Williams
Obstetrics

20th Edition

This study guide includes continuing medical education material, an educational activity sponsored by:

SOUTHWESTERN

THE UNIVERSITY OF TEXAS
SOUTHWESTERN MEDICAL CENTER
AT DALLAS

ACCME Accreditation

The University of Texas Southwestern Medical Center at Dallas is accredited by the Accreditation Council for Continuing Medical Education to sponsor continuing medical education for physicians.

AMA/PRA Credit Designation

The University of Texas Southwestern Medical Center at Dallas designates this educational activity for a maximum of 50 hours in Category I credit towards the AMA Physician's Recognition Award. Each physician should claim only those hours of credit that he or she actually spent in the educational activity.

This CME activity was planned and produced in accordance with the ACCME Essentials.
Date of original release: December 1996; Term of approval: 3 years

See page 261 for additional CME instructions.

The University of Texas Southwestern Medical Center at Dallas Office of Continuing Education

DISCLOSURE OF SIGNIFICANT RELATIONSHIPS WITH RELEVANT COMMERCIAL COMPANIES/ORGANIZATIONS

Study Guide for Williams Obstetrics, 20th Edition
December 1996

According to the University of Texas Southwestern "Disclosure Policy," faculty involved in continuing medical education activities are required to complete a "Conflict of Interest Disclosure" to disclose any real or apparent conflict(s) of interest related directly or indirectly to the program. This information is acknowledged solely for the information of the participant.

The faculty listed below have disclosed a financial interest or other relationship with a commercial concern related directly or indirectly to the activity (names of companies are listed after each presenter's name). Those presenters not listed have disclosed no financial interest or relationship.

UT Southwestern does not view the existence of these interests or relationships as implying bias or decreasing the value of the presentation.

This educational activity has been planned to be well-balanced and objective in discussion of comparative treatment regimens. Information and opinions offered by the authors represent their viewpoints. Conclusions drawn by the reader should be derived from careful consideration of all available scientific information. Products may be discussed in treatment of indications outside current approved labeling.

Faculty

Larry C. Gilstrap III, MD	Author of *Study Guide for Williams Obstetrics, 20th Edition*, 1996
Susan B. Cox, MD	Author of *Study Guide for Williams Obstetrics, 20th Edition*, 1996
Alvin L. Brekken, MD	Author of *Study Guide for Williams Obstetrics, 20th Edition*, 1996
F. Gary Cunningham, MD	Author of *Study Guide for Williams Obstetrics, 20th Edition*, 1996

Study Guide for

Williams Obstetrics

20th Edition

Larry C. Gilstrap III, MD
Professor and Chairman
Department of Obstetrics & Gynecology
University of Texas Medical School at Houston
Houston, Texas
Formerly
Professor
Department of Obstetrics & Gynecology
The University of Texas Southwestern Medical
  Center at Dallas
Dallas, Texas

Susan M. Cox, MD
Associate Professor
Department of Obstetrics & Gynecology
The University of Texas Southwestern Medical
  Center at Dallas
Dallas, Texas

Alvin L. Brekken, MD
Professor and Vice Chairman
Department of Obstetrics & Gynecology
The University of Texas Southwestern Medical
  Center at Dallas
Dallas, Texas

F. Gary Cunningham, MD
Professor and Chairman
Department of Obstetrics & Gynecology
Jack A. Pritchard Professor of Obstetrics & Gynecology
Beatrice & Miguel Elias Distinguished Chair in
  Obstetrics & Gynecology
The University of Texas Southwestern Medical
  Center at Dallas
Chief of Obstetrics & Gynecology
Parkland Memorial Hospital
Dallas, Texas

Instructions for obtaining CME credit appear on page 261.

APPLETON & LANGE
Stamford, Connecticut

97 98 99 00 01/10 9 8 7 6 5 4 3 2 1

Prentice Hall International (UK) Limited, *London*
Prentice Hall of Australia Pty. Limited, *Sydney*
Prentice Hall Canada, Inc., *Toronto*
Prentice Hall Hispanoamericana, S.A., *Mexico*
Prentice Hall of India Private Limited, *New Delhi*
Prentice Hall of Japan, Inc., *Tokyo*
Simon and Schuster Asia Pte. Ltd., *Singapore*
Editora Prentice Hall do Brasil Ltda., *Rio de Janeiro*
Prentice Hall, *Upper Saddle River, New Jersey*

Acquisitions Editor: Jane Licht
Production Editor: Eileen Pendagast
Production Service: Spectrum Publisher Services
Cover Designer: Mary Skudlarek

ISBN 0-8385-9641-X

90000

9 780838 596418

PRINTED IN THE UNITED STATES OF AMERICA

Contents

Preface

This *Study Guide for Williams Obstetrics* is designed to assess comprehension and retention of materials covered in the 20th edition of *Williams Obstetrics*. A new feature of this study guide is the provision for earning continuing medical education (CME) credit.

The questions for each section are based on the key points from each chapter and are in the same order as the text. There are over 2000 questions from the 62 chapters. The questions are in multiple choice format. It is suggested that the reader read the question and think of the answer prior to choosing the single most correct answer from the four choices provided. The questions are followed by a section that contains the answers and page numbers in the textbook where the answers can be found.

We hope that the simplified format used in this study guide will make the task of assimilating the information from the 20th edition of *Williams Obstetrics* less formidable. It is also hoped that the provision for earning CME credit will lend itself to the extremely busy, everyday practice of clinical medicine.

Larry C. Gilstrap III, MD
Susan M. Cox, MD
Alvin L. Brekken, MD
F. Gary Cunningham, MD

HUMAN PREGNANCY

1

Obstetrics in Broad Perspective

1–1. The word *obstetrics* is derived from the Latin term *obstetrix,* which means which of the following?

    a. midwife
    b. deliverer
    c. attendant
    d. surgeon

1–2. What year was the Bureau of the Census established?

    a. 1858
    b. 1902
    c. 1928
    d. 1952

1–3. Which of one of the following corresponds to the perinatal period?

    a. 22 to 28 weeks gestation
    b. 22 to 34 weeks gestation
    c. 20 to 40 weeks gestation
    d. 20 weeks to 4 weeks postpartum

1–4. Which of the following describes the number of live births per 1000 population?

    a. fertility rate
    b. birth rate
    c. live birth rate
    d. delivery rate

1–5. What is the number of deaths per 1000 births occurring during the first 28 days of life?

    a. stillbirth rate
    b. fetal death rate
    c. perinatal mortality rate
    d. neonatal mortality rate

1–6. What is the upper gestational age cutoff for defining the birth of a preterm infant?

    a. 29 weeks
    b. 33 weeks
    c. 35 weeks
    d. 37 weeks

1–7. How would a maternal death secondary to mitral stenosis be classified?

  a. a direct maternal death
  b. an indirect maternal death
  c. a nonmaternal death
  d. a nonobstetrical death

1–8. How is an infant classified that is born between 260 and 294 days of gestation?

  a. preterm infant
  b. term infant
  c. postterm infant
  d. postmature infant

1–9. What was the maternal mortality rate for the United States in 1994?

  a. 1.1 per 100,000 live births
  b. 4.6 per 100,000 live births
  c. 8.5 per 100,000 live births
  d. 15.1 per 100,000 live births

1–10. What is the single most common cause of maternal mortality?

  a. embolism
  b. hypertension
  c. hemorrhage
  d. ectopic pregnancy

1–11. What percentage of perinatal deaths are stillbirths?

  a. 10
  b. 25
  c. 50
  d. 75

1–12. What is the single most common cause of neonatal death?

  a. low birthweight
  b. congenital anomalies
  c. infection
  d. perinatal asphyxia

1–13. How is the neonatal death rate expressed?

  a. per 1000 live births
  b. per 10,000 live births
  c. per 100,000 live births
  d. per 1,000,000 live births

1–14. What was the perinatal mortality rate for the United States in 1991?

  a. 5.0 per 1000
  b. 7.0 per 1000
  c. 12.8 per 1000
  d. 16.8 per 1000

1–15. What is the leading cause of death in black women aged 25 to 44 years?

  a. accident
  b. suicide
  c. human immunodeficiency virus infection
  d. thromboembolism

1–16. Which of the following is NOT a result of the "litigation crisis"?

  a. a decrease in the availability of obstetrical care for indigent women
  b. an increase in the number of skilled clinicians retiring from obstetrics
  c. an increase in the cost of care
  d. a decrease in the frequency of cerebral palsy

2

Pregnancy: Overview and Diagnosis

2–1. In a woman who does not use contraception, how many lifetime opportunities are there for pregnancy?

   a. 100
   b. 250
   c. 500
   d. 1000

2–2. What percentage of married couples have relative or absolute infertility?

   a. 1
   b. 5
   c. 10
   d. 20

2–3. What is the approximate success of in vitro fertilization and embryo transfer in producing a live-born fetus?

   a. 12 percent
   b. 25 percent
   c. 41 percent
   d. 65 percent

2–4. How many generations have there been since the birth of Christ?

   a. 10
   b. 20
   c. 40
   d. 80

2–5. Which of the following mammals does not menstruate?

   a. old world monkeys
   b. dolphins
   c. great apes
   d. chimpanzees

2–6. What is the average age of menarche for women in the United States?

   a. $11\frac{1}{2}$ years
   b. $12\frac{1}{2}$ years
   c. $13\frac{1}{2}$ years
   d. $14\frac{1}{2}$ years

2–7. What is the site of synthesis of follicular estrogen?

   a. granulosa cells
   b. theca cells
   c. stroma cells
   d. endometrium

2–8. Which of the following is NOT a component of the paracrine arm of the fetal–maternal communication system?

   a. pregnancy maintenance
   b. immunological acceptance
   c. amnionic fluid volume homeostasis
   d. endocrine processes

2–9. How is human placentation described?

   a. epitheliochorial
   b. hemochorioendothelial
   c. endotheliochorial
   d. hemoendothelial

2–10. Which of the following hormones is produced by the decidua?

   a. prolactin
   b. estrogen
   c. prostaglandin F_2
   d. progesterone

2–11. Which of the following is a vasoconstrictor produced by the amnion?

    a. parathyroid hormone-related protein
    b. endothelin-1
    c. prostaglandin I_2
    d. thromboxane

2–12. How long after fertilization does it take for the zygote to reach the uterine cavity?

    a. 1 to 2 days
    b. 3 to 4 days
    c. 5 to 6 days
    d. 7 days

2–13. What hormone is responsible for maintenance of the corpus luteum if implantation of the fertilized ovum takes place?

    a. estrogen
    b. progesterone
    c. hCG
    d. hPL

2–14. What hormone is responsible for rescuing the corpus luteum of menstruation?

    a. estradiol
    b. human chorionic gonadotropin (hCG)
    c. progesterone
    d. human placental lactogen (hPL)

2–15. At what menstrual age (weeks) does progesterone synthesis in the syncytiotrophoblast become dominant?

    a. 2
    b. 4
    c. 6
    d. 8

2–16. Which of the following hormones acts to prevent lactogenesis?

    a. human placental lactogen (hPL)
    b. prolactin
    c. cortisol
    d. progesterone

2–17. Which of the following is NOT a presumptive symptom of pregnancy?

    a. nausea
    b. fatigue
    c. urinary frequency
    d. constipation

2–18. Which of the following is NOT a positive sign of pregnancy?

    a. identification of fetal heart tones
    b. positive pregnancy test
    c. perception of fetal movement by examiner
    d. identification of fetus by sonography

2–19. What percentage of pregnancies that do not abort are associated with macroscopic vaginal bleeding?

    a. <5%
    b. 20 to 25%
    c. 50 to 60%
    d. 80 to 90%

2–20. What is the Chadwick sign?

    a. discoloration of the vaginal mucosa
    b. pigmentation of the skin
    c. change in consistency of uterus
    d. implantation bleeding

2–21. Which of the following is NOT considered a probable sign of pregnancy?

    a. enlargement of the abdomen
    b. changes in shape, size, and consistency of uterus
    c. cessation of menses
    d. ballottement

2–22. How long after onset of last menstruation until Hegar sign becomes evident?

    a. <1 week
    b. 2 to 4 weeks
    c. 6 to 8 weeks
    d. >10 weeks

2–23. What is the earliest time following ovulation that human chorionic gonadotropin can be detected in maternal urine or plasma?

    a. 5 to 6 days
    b. 8 to 9 days
    c. 10 to 12 days
    d. 14 to 16 days

2–24. What is the doubling time for human chorionic gonadotropin in early pregnancy?

    a. 1.5 to 2.0 days
    b. 2.5 to 3.0 days

c. 4.5 to 5.0 days
d. >5.0 days

2–25. What is the sensitivity of the enzyme-linked immunosorbent assay (ELISA) test for human chorionic gonadotropin?

a. 10 mIU/mL
b. 20 mIU/mL
c. 50 mIU/mL
d. 250 mIU/mL

2–26. A "normal" doubling of human chorionic gonadotropin is associated with a successful pregnancy outcome in what percentage of cases?

a. 50
b. 65
c. 75
d. 90

2–27. A normal doubling time of human chorionic gonadotropin is found in what percentage of ectopic pregnancies?

a. <1
b. 5
c. 20
d. 50

2–28. What is the sound caused by the rush of blood through the umbilical arteries called?

a. funic souffle
b. fetal souffle
c. placental souffle
d. uterine souffle

2–29. The "white gestational ring" can first be identified at what age?

a. 4 weeks
b. 5 weeks
c. 6 weeks
d. 8 weeks

2–30. Up to what gestational age is the crown–rump length predictive of gestational age within 4 days?

a. 8 weeks
b. 10 weeks

c. 12 weeks
d. 14 weeks

2–31. Which of the following is NOT a characteristic feature of blighted ovum?

a. small white gestational ring is identified
b. loss of definition of gestational sac
c. unusually small gestational sac
d. no fetal echoes

2–32. The fetal head and thorax can first be identified at what gestational age?

a. 9 to 10 weeks
b. 11 to 12 weeks
c. 13 to 14 weeks
d. 15 weeks

2–33. By utilizing vaginal sonography, how early after conception can the chorionic cavity be identified?

a. 2 weeks
b. 3 weeks
c. 4 weeks
d. 5 weeks

2–34. The fetal skeleton can usually not be identified radiographically until what gestational age?

a. 12 weeks
b. 14 weeks
c. 16 weeks
d. 18 weeks

2–35. Which of the following radiographic signs signifies fetal death?

a. straightened fetal spine
b. areas of gas in the fetus
c. overlapping skull bones (Spalding sign)
d. gas in the amnionic fluid

2–36. 17α-Hydroxyprogesterone (150 mg intramuscularly) is recommended when the corpus luteum is removed prior to what week of gestation?

a. 10
b. 12
c. 16
d. 20

3

Anatomy of the Reproductive Tract

3–1. The labia majora are homologous with which of the following male structures?

   a. glans penis
   b. scrotum
   c. gubernaculum testis
   d. corpora cavernosa

3–2. The labia minora are covered by which of the following structures?

   a. mucous membrane
   b. hair
   c. transitional epithelium
   d. stratified squamous epithelium

3–3. The clitoris is the homologue of which of the following structures?

   a. penis
   b. scrotum
   c. gubernaculum testis
   d. corpora cavernosa

3–4. What is the principal erogenous organ or area of women?

   a. vagina
   b. clitoris
   c. labia minora
   d. G-spot

3–5. Embryologically, the vestibular bulbs correspond to which of the following male anlages?

   a. corpora cavernosa of the penis
   b. corpora spongiosa of the penis
   c. dorsal vein of the penis
   d. testicular venous plexus

3–6. Which of the following is the predominant bacteria of the vagina during pregnancy?

   a. *Peptostreptococcus* sp.
   b. *Listeria monocytogenes*

   c. *Lactobacillus* sp.
   d. *Streptococcus agalactiae*

3–7. What portion of the vagina is formed from the Müllerian ducts?

   a. upper portion
   b. middle portion
   c. lower portion
   d. hymenal portion

3–8. The urogenital sinus gives rise to what portion of the vagina?

   a. upper portion
   b. middle portion
   c. lower portion
   d. hymenal portion

3–9. What is the pH range of vaginal secretions before puberty?

   a. 2.0 to 3.4
   b. 3.6 to 4.2
   c. 4.0 to 5.0
   d. 6.8 to 7.2

3–10. What is the blood supply to the upper third of the vagina?

   a. cervicovaginal branch of the uterine artery
   b. inferior vesical arteries
   c. superior vesical arteries
   d. rectal and internal pudendal arteries

3–11. What is the blood supply of the middle third of the vagina?

   a. cervicovaginal branch of the uterine artery
   b. inferior vesical arteries
   c. superior vesical arteries
   d. rectal and internal pudendal arteries

3–12. What is the blood supply of the lower third of the vagina?

    a. cervicovaginal branch of the uterine artery

    b. inferior vesical arteries

    c. superior vesical arteries

    d. middle rectal and internal pudendal arteries

3–13. Which artery below is a branch of the internal pudendal artery?

    a. inferior vesical artery

    b. cervicovaginal artery

    c. superior rectal artery

    d. posterior labial artery

3–14. What is the origin of the pudendal nerve?

    a. L4-5, S1-2

    b. S1-3

    c. S2-4

    d. S4-5

3–15. What is the average weight of a nulliparous adult uterus?

    a. 20 to 30 g

    b. 50 to 70 g

    c. 80 to 90 g

    d. 100 to 150 g

3–16. What is the average length of a parous uterus?

    a. 2.5 to 3.5 cm

    b. 4 to 6 cm

    c. 6 to 8 cm

    d. 9 to 10 cm

3–17. What is the total volume of the uterus at term?

    a. 2.5 L

    b. 3.5 L

    c. 5.0 L

    d. 7.0 L

3–18. Approximately what percentage of the normal cervix is composed of muscle?

    a. <1

    b. 10

    c. 25

    d. 50

3–19. Which of the following arteries penetrates the middle third of the uterine wall and runs in a plane parallel to the uterine surface?

    a. arcuate

    b. radial

    c. basal

    d. coiled

3–20. The uterine artery is a main branch of which of the following arteries?

    a. aorta

    b. common iliac

    c. external iliac

    d. internal iliac

3–21. The uterine artery most commonly crosses over the ureter at which of the following locations?

    a. 1.0 cm lateral to the cervix

    b. 2.0 cm lateral to the cervix

    c. 3.5 cm lateral to the cervix

    d. 4.5 cm lateral to the cervix

3–22. The ovarian artery is a direct branch of which of the following vessels?

    a. aorta

    b. common iliac

    c. external iliac

    d. internal iliac

3–23. Which of the following nerve roots provide sensory fibers from the uterus that are associated with the painful stimuli of uterine contractions?

    a. T-9 and T-10

    b. T-11 and T-12

    c. L-1 and L-2

    d. S-2, S-3, and S-4

3–24. What is the single layer of cuboidal epithelium on the surface of the ovary?

    a. tunica albuginea

    b. germinal epithelium of Waldeyer

    c. the primordial layer of wolffian

    d. tunica cortex

3–25. What is the estimated number of oocytes at puberty?

   a. 50,000 to 100,000
   b. 200,000 to 400,000
   c. 750,000 to 1 million
   d. 3 to 5 million

3–26. Gartner duct cysts are remnants of which of the following?

   a. mesonephric duct
   b. paramesonephric duct
   c. metanephric duct
   d. parametanephric duct

3–27. Which of the following is NOT a component of the bony pelvis?

   a. coccyx
   b. sacrum
   c. ischium
   d. femoral head

3–28. Which of the following is NOT part of the superior boundary of the true pelvis?

   a. linea terminalis
   b. lumbar vertebrae
   c. promontory of the sacrum
   d. pubic bones

3–29. The true pelvis is bounded below by which of the following structures?

   a. sacral promontory
   b. alae of sacral
   c. pelvic outlet
   d. upper margins of pelvic bone

3–30. What is the shortest diameter of the pelvic cavity?

   a. diagonal conjugate
   b. interspinous
   c. true conjugate
   d. obstetrical conjugate

3–31. What are the results of a modified squatting position in the second stage of labor?

   a. a longer second stage
   b. more perineal lacerations
   c. more labial lacerations
   d. less caput and molding

3–32. Which of the following is NOT one of the four imaginary planes of the pelvis?

   a. superior strait
   b. inferior strait
   c. least pelvic dimensions
   d. lateral straits

3–33. What is the average transverse diameter of the pelvic inlet?

   a. 8.0 cm
   b. 10.0 cm
   c. 10.5 cm
   d. 13.5 cm

3–34. What is the average interspinous diameter?

   a. 8.0 cm
   b. 10.0 cm
   c. 10.5 cm
   d. 12.0 cm

3–35. What is the average diameter of the obstetrical conjugate?

   a. 8.0 cm
   b. 10.0 cm
   c. 10.5 cm
   d. 12.0 cm

3–36. What is the average transverse diameter of the pelvic outlet?

   a. 8.0 cm
   b. 10.0 cm
   c. 10.5 cm
   d. 11.0 cm

3–37. Which of the following best describes the anterior pelvis that is narrow, with convergent sidewalls, prominent ischial spines, and a narrow subpubic arch?

   a. gynecoid
   b. android
   c. anthropoid
   d. platypelloid

3–38. What type of pelvis is characterized by a short anterior-posterior diameter and a wide transverse diameter?

   a. gynecoid
   b. android
   c. anthropoid
   d. platypelloid

3–39. What type of pelvis is associated with an inlet that is round, with straight pelvic sidewalls, spines that are not prominent, and a wide pelvic arch?

    a. gynecoid
    b. android
    c. anthropoid
    d. platypelloid

3–40. The anthropoid pelvis type is found in what percentage of white women?

    a. 3
    b. 10
    c. 25
    d. 33

3–41. What percentage of white women have an android-type pelvis?

    a. 3
    b. 10
    c. 25
    d. 33

3–42. What percentage of nonwhite women have an anthropoid-type pelvis?

    a. 3
    b. 12
    c. 25
    d. 50

3–43. How is the obstetrical conjugate computed?

    a. add 1.5 cm to the diagonal conjugate
    b. subtract 1.5 cm from the diagonal conjugate
    c. average the diagonal and true conjugate measures
    d. add 1.5 cm to the true conjugate

3–44. What is the approximate distance from the plane of the pelvic inlet to the level of the ischial spines?

    a. 1 cm
    b. 2 cm
    c. 3 cm
    d. 5 cm

3–45. What is the distance from the biparietal plane of the unmolded fetal head to the vertex?

    a. <1 cm
    b. 1 to 2 cm
    c. 3 to 4 cm
    d. 6 to 8 cm

3–46. What is descent of the fetal head through the pelvic inlet to a depth that prevents its free movement called?

    a. engagement
    b. fixation
    c. station
    d. adaption

3–47. What anatomical structure separates the true from the false pelvis?

    a. lumbar vertebrae
    b. anterior abdominal wall
    c. ischial spines
    d. linea terminalis

3–48. Which of the following is NOT involved in the anterior junction of the pelvic bones?

    a. superior pubic ligament
    b. inferior pubic ligament
    c. sacroiliac joint
    d. symphysis pubis

Physiology of Pregnancy

$$\boxed{4}$$

The Endometrium and Decidua: Menstruation and Pregnancy

4–1. What does the portion of the decidua invaded by the trophoblast become?

    a. decidua basalis
    b. decidua capsularis
    c. decidua vera
    d. decidua parietalis

4–2. Which of the following is NOT produced by the decidua?

    a. 1,25-dihydroxy-vitamin-D_3
    b. corticotropin-releasing hormone
    c. relaxin
    d. thyroid-stimulating hormone

4–3. Where is the primary location for sex hormone steroid receptors (i.e., estradiol, etc.)?

    a. cytoplasm (i.e., "cytosol preparation")
    b. cell membrane
    c. messenger RNA
    d. nucleus

4–4. Which of the following best describes the receptors for estradiol and progesterone?

    a. high affinity, low capacity
    b. high affinity, high capacity
    c. low affinity, low capacity
    d. low affinity, high capacity

4–5. As an antiestrogen, progesterone does NOT attenuate the action of estrogen by which of the following mechanisms?

    a. decreases estrogen receptors
    b. displaces estrogen from receptors
    c. increases estradiol dehydrogenase
    d. increases sulfurylation of estrogens

4–6. Re-epithelialization resulting in the epithelial surface of the endometrium being restored is complete by which day of the endometrial cycle?

    a. 2
    b. 5
    c. 8
    d. 12

4–7. Infiltration of the stroma by polymorphonuclear and mononuclear leukocytes occurs in what part of the menstrual cycle?

    a. late proliferative phase
    b. early secretory phase
    c. midsecretory phase
    d. premenstrual phase

4–8. Which of the following substances is associated with the intense vasoconstriction of the spiral arteries that begins 4 to 24 hours before onset of bleeding?

    a. interleukin-8
    b. monocyte peptide-1
    c. prostaglandin E_2
    d. endothelin-1

4–9. Which of the following enzymes serves to degrade a number of highly bioactive peptides such as atrial natriuretic peptide, substance P, and endothelin-1?

    a. enkephalinase
    b. phospholipase A_2
    c. prostaglandin dehydrogenase
    d. phospholipase C

4–10. Which of the following is NOT produced by endometrial stromal cells?

    a. endothelin-1
    b. enkephalinase
    c. parathyroid hormone-related protein (PTH-rP)
    d. 15-hydroxyprostaglandin dehydrogenase (PGDH)

4–11. What day of the menstrual cycle do subnuclear, glycogen-rich vacuoles develop in the glandular epithelium?

    a. 5 to 7
    b. 10 to 12
    c. 14 to 16
    d. 20 to 22

4–12. What is the average age of menarche for women living in the United States?

    a. 9 to 10
    b. 11
    c. 12 to 13
    d. 14 to 15

4–13. Approximately what percentage of a woman's cycles will vary more than 2 days from the mean of the length of her cycles?

    a. <1
    b. 5
    c. 33
    d. 50

4–14. What is the average amount of blood lost during a normal menstrual cycle?

    a. 10 to 15 mL
    b. 25 to 60 mL
    c. 85 to 120 mL
    d. 150 mL

4–15. The renaissance in anatomy can be attributed to which of the following?

    a. da Vinci
    b. dei Luzzi
    c. Vesalius
    d. Paracelsus

4–16. What is the most likely explanation for the premenstrual syndrome (PMS)?

    a. massive estrogen secretion
    b. massive progesterone secretion
    c. massive prostaglandin secretion
    d. massive endothelin secretion

4–17. What is estramedin?

    a. a synonym for estrogen
    b. an antagonist of progesterone
    c. a growth factor
    d. essential in the initiation of menses

4–18. At what week of gestation is the uterine cavity obliterated by the fusion of the decidua capsularis and parietalis?

    a. 6 to 8
    b. 10 to 13
    c. 14 to 16
    d. 18 to 20

4–19. Which of the following is defective or absent in the case of placenta accreta?

    a. decidua basalis
    b. Nitabuch's layer
    c. Rohr's stria
    d. decidual stromal cells

4–20. In the midluteal phase of the menstrual cycle, how much progesterone is produced per day?

    a. 40 to 50 μg
    b. 40 to 50 mg
    c. 40 to 50 grams
    d. none of the above

4–21. What is the duration of the luteal phase of the menstrual cycle?

    a. variable
    b. 10 to 12 days
    c. 12 to 14 days
    d. most commonly over 14 days

4–22. What is the duration of the proliferative phase of the menstrual cycle?

    a. variable
    b. 10 to 12 days
    c. 12 to 14 days
    d. most commonly over 14 days

4–23. Of the following, which causes vasoconstriction of the spinal arterioles?

    a. PGI_2
    b. nitric acid
    c. endothelin
    d. enkephalinase

The Placenta and Fetal Membranes

5–1. What is the solid ball of cells formed by 16 or more blastomeres?

    a. morula
    b. blastocyst
    c. zygote
    d. embryo

5–2. Up until the end of the 7th week, what term is used to describe the product of conception?

    a. zygote
    b. embryo
    c. fetus
    d. conceptus

5–3. At what stage of development does the conceptus implant?

    a. zygote
    b. morula

    c. blastocyst
    d. embryo

5–4. What is the most common uterine site for implantation in the human?

    a. upper posterior wall
    b. lower posterior wall
    c. upper anterior wall
    d. lower anterior wall

5–5. What is the origin of the syncytiotrophoblast?

    a. inner cell mass
    b. cytotrophoblast
    c. zona pellucida
    d. decidua capsularis

5–6. Which of the following statements is NOT true regarding the hemochorioendothelial placenta?

   a. It is the type of placenta found in most animals.
   b. Maternal blood directly bathes the syncytiotrophoblast.
   c. Fetal blood is separated from maternal blood.
   d. At all sites of direct contact, maternal tissue is juxtaposed to fetal trophoblast and not embryonic cells.

5–7. The term *conceptus* includes all but which of the following?

   a. embryo
   b. fetal membranes
   c. decidua
   d. placenta

5–8. Pregnancy is least likely to occur if coitus occurs at which time?

   a. at ovulation
   b. 2 days after ovulation
   c. 2 days before ovulation
   d. 1 day before ovulation

5–9. The survival of the conceptus in the uterus is attributable to the immunological peculiarity of which of the following?

   a. decidua
   b. amnion
   c. chorion
   d. trophoblast

5–10. What is the average length of the umbilical cord?

   a. 30 cm
   b. 55 cm
   c. 80 cm
   d. 100 cm

5–11. When is a true placental circulation established?

   a. 12th day after fertilization
   b. 14th day after fertilization
   c. 17th day after fertilization
   d. 28th day after fertilization

5–12. What do the villi in contact with the decidua basalis proliferate to form?

   a. chorion frondosum
   b. chorion laeve
   c. chorion basalis
   d. chorion capsularis

5–13. What are a main stem (truncal) villi and its ramifications?

   a. placental cotyledon
   b. maternal cotyledon
   c. stem cotyledon
   d. primary cotyledon

5–14. What is the average volume of the term placenta?

   a. 100 mL
   b. 300 mL
   c. 500 mL
   d. 750 mL

5–15. What are fetal macrophages found in the stroma of villi?

   a. Hofbauer cells
   b. Langhan cells
   c. K-cells
   d. septal cells

5–16. Which of the following changes are NOT associated with placental aging?

   a. a decrease in thickness of syncytium
   b. an increase in Langhans cells
   c. a decrease in stroma
   d. an increase in number of capillaries

5–17. Leukocytes bearing a Y chromosome have been identified in women for how long after giving birth to a son?

   a. 6 months
   b. 1 year
   c. 2 years
   d. 5 years

5–18. Class II major histocompatibility complex (MHC) antigens are absent from trophoblasts at what stage of gestation?

   a. first trimester
   b. second trimester
   c. third trimester
   d. at all stages

5–19. How many spiral arterial entries into the intervillous space are present at term?

    a. 30
    b. 50
    c. 80
    d. 120

5–20. Who first described the physiological mechanism of placental circulation?

    a. Ramsey
    b. Benirschke
    c. Bleker
    d. Harvey

5–21. What term describes the persistence of the intra-abdominal portion of the duct of the umbilical vessels, which extends from the umbilicus to the intestine?

    a. allantoic remnant
    b. duct of Hoboken
    c. Meckel diverticulum
    d. omphalocele

6

The Placental Hormones

6–1. Which of the following is NOT an example of chemical characteristics of human chorionic gonadotropin (hCG)?

    a. glycoprotein
    b. highest carbohydrate content of any human hormone
    c. both α- and β-subunits are necessary for bioactivity
    d. the β-subunit is most closely related to the β-subunit of FSH

6–2. All eight of the genes for the β-subunit of human chorionic gonadotropin are located on which of the following chromosomes?

    a. 1
    b. 9
    c. 19
    d. X

6–3. Where is the complete molecule of human chorionic gonadotropin primarily produced?

    a. syncytiotrophoblast
    b. cytotrophoblast

    c. chorioamnionic membrane
    d. Hofbauer cells

6–4. The maximum levels of human chorionic gonadotropin in maternal serum occur at what week of pregnancy?

    a. 4th
    b. 10th
    c. 16th
    d. 20th

6–5. The nadir in the level of human chorionic gonadotropin in maternal serum is reached at what week of pregnancy?

    a. 6th
    b. 10th
    c. 16th
    d. 20th

6–6. What is the average peak level of human chorionic gonadotropin in maternal serum during normal pregnancy?

    a. 1 IU/mL
    b. 10 IU/mL
    c. 100 IU/mL
    d. 1000 IU/mL

6–7. Which of the following regarding the nicks in the human chorionic gonadotropin molecule is NOT true?

   a. They occur mainly in the β-subunit amino acids.

   b. Their origin is most likely attributable to enzymatic action.

   c. Their biological importance is unknown.

   d. The immunoreactivity to monoclonal antibodies is unaffected by nicks.

6–8. What is the best known function of human chorionic gonadotropin?

   a. its maintenance of the corpus luteum

   b. that it helps protect against paternal antibodies

   c. that it stimulates human placental lactogen secretion

   d. that it stimulates fetal ovaries to produce estrogen

6–9. What is the half-life of human chorionic gonadotropin?

   a. 30 min

   b. 4 hr

   c. 24 hr

   d. 36 hr

6–10. Regarding the chemical characteristics of human placental lactogen, which of the following is most correct?

   a. molecular weight is 150,000

   b. contains 191 amino acids

   c. amino acids have 94 percent homology with human growth hormone

   d. is most similar to human prolactin

6–11. When (week of pregnancy) does human placental lactogen peak in the maternal serum?

   a. 10th to 12th

   b. 16th to 20th

   c. 28th to 30th

   d. 34th to 36th

6–12. What is the half-life of human placental lactogen?

   a. 30 min

   b. 6 hr

   c. 12 hr

   d. 36 hr

6–13. Which of the following is NOT an action of human placental lactogen?

   a. lipolysis

   b. anti-insulin action

   c. stimulate protein synthesis

   d. stimulates fetal testes to produce testosterone

6–14. Which of the following is NOT derived from the precursor molecule, pro-opiomelanocortin (POMC)?

   a. human placental lactogen (hPL)

   b. corticotropin (ACTH)

   c. lipoprotein

   d. β-endorphin

6–15. Which of the following is most likely responsible for the increased thyroid-stimulating activity in women with neoplastic trophoblastic disease?

   a. chorionic thyrotropin (hCT)

   b. human placental lactogen (hPL)

   c. human chorionic gonadotropin (hCG)

   d. corticotropin-releasing hormone (CRH)

6–16. What is the probable role of placental inhibin?

   a. suppresses the follicle-stimulating hormone (FSH)

   b. suppresses the thyroxine-releasing hormone (TRH)

   c. suppresses the gonadotropin-releasing hormone (GnRH)

   d. suppresses the corticotropin-releasing hormone (CRH)

6–17. What is a precursor for estrogen biosynthesis in the human placenta?

   a. acetate

   b. cholesterol

   c. progesterone

   d. dehydroepiandrosterone sulfate

6–18. What is the quantitatively important source of placental estrogen precursor in the human?

   a. maternal adrenal

   b. syncytiotrophoblast

   c. cytotrophoblast

   d. fetal adrenal

6–19. The fetus is the source of approximately what percentage of the precursor of the estriol formed in the placenta?

   a. 5
   b. 25
   c. 50
   d. 90

6–20. Approximately what percentage of the fetal adrenal is composed of the fetal zone?

   a. 5
   b. 25
   c. 55
   d. 85

6–21. Relative to body weight, how much larger are the adrenals of the human fetus at term than those of the adult?

   a. 2 times
   b. 10 times
   c. 25 times
   d. 50 times

6–22. What is the precursor used for steroid biosynthesis in the fetal adrenal?

   a. cholesterol
   b. acetate
   c. progesterone
   d. pregnenolone

6–23. What is the major source of fetal plasma LDL-cholesterol?

   a. maternal transfer
   b. placental synthesis
   c. fetal liver
   d. fetal adrenal

6–24. What happens to umbilical cord plasma levels of estrogens and progesterone in infants of women with pregnancy-induced hypertension, chronic hypertension, and severe forms of diabetes mellitus compared with infants of normal women?

   a. increases slightly
   b. increases significantly
   c. decreases slightly
   d. decreases significantly

6–25. What is the placental enzyme that "protects" the female fetus from virilization in a pregnant woman with an androgen-secreting ovarian tumor?

   a. aromatase
   b. sulfatase
   c. 17α-hydroxylase
   d. 3β-hydroxysteroid dehydrogenase

6–26. Placental sulfatase deficiency (also associated with ichthyosis) is what type of disorder?

   a. multifactorial
   b. X-linked recessive
   c. autosomal dominant
   d. autosomal recessive

6–27. What is the precursor for the biosynthesis of progesterone by the placenta?

   a. placental actetate
   b. maternal LDL-cholesterol
   c. fetal pregnenolone
   d. fetal C-19 steroids

6–28. What is the approximate daily production of progesterone in late normal, singleton pregnancies?

   a. 50 mg
   b. 250 mg
   c. 1200 mg
   d. 2400 mg

6–29. What is the cause of the marked increase in the potent mineralocorticosteroid, deoxycorticosterone, seen in pregnancy?

   a. increased fetal adrenal production
   b. increased maternal adrenal production
   c. increased placental production
   d. extra-adrenal conversion of progesterone

7

The Morphological and Functional Development of the Fetus

7–1. Pregnancy is said to consist of 10 lunar months. How long is an actual lunar month?

    a. 26 days
    b. 27 days
    c. 28 days
    d. 29 days

7–2. What are the products of conception known as prior to implantation?

    a. a zygote
    b. pregnancy products
    c. a conceptus
    d. a fetus

7–3. Which of the following best represents the embryonic period?

    a. fertilization to 6 weeks
    b. implantation to 6 weeks
    c. 3rd to 8th week after fertilization
    d. first 11 to 12 weeks of pregnancy

7–4. What is the approximate crown–rump length of the fetus by the end of the 12th week of pregnancy?

    a. 1 to 2 cm
    b. 4 cm
    c. 6 to 7 cm
    d. 12 cm

7–5. What is the approximate weight of the fetus at 16 gestational weeks?

    a. 25 g
    b. 50 g
    c. 110 g
    d. 250 g

7–6. What is the approximate weight of the fetus at 20 gestational weeks?

    a. 200 g
    b. 300 g
    c. 480 g
    d. 650 g

7–7. What is the approximate weight of the fetus at 24 gestational weeks?

    a. 500 g
    b. 630 g
    c. 750 g
    d. 890 g

7–8. What is the approximate weight of the fetus at 28 gestational weeks?

    a. 750 g
    b. 890 g
    c. 1100 g
    d. 1500 g

7–9. What is the average weight of the fetus at 32 gestational weeks?

    a. 1000 g
    b. 1500 g
    c. 1800 g
    d. 2000 g

7–10. What is the average weight of the fetus at 36 gestational weeks?

    a. 1990 g
    b. 2500 g
    c. 2850 g
    d. 3000 g

7–11. What is the largest baby recorded in the medical literature (a stillborn female)?

a. 14.0 lb
b. 16.5 lb
c. 18.0 lb
d. 25.0 lb

7–12. In the fetus or neonate, what are the two sutures between the posterior margin of the parietal bones and the upper margin of the occipital bone called?

a. occipitalis
b. sagittal
c. lambdoid
d. coronal

7–13. In the fetus or neonate, what are the two sutures between the frontal and parietal bones?

a. frontal
b. sagittal
c. lambdoid
d. coronal

7–14. Which of the following diameters has the greatest length?

a. occipitofrontal
b. biparietal
c. occipitomental
d. suboccipitobregmatic

7–15. The plane of which of the following diameters represents the greatest circumference of the head?

a. occipitofrontal
b. suboccipitobregmatic
c. bitemporal
d. biparietal

7–16. The plane of which of the following diameters represents the smallest circumference of the head?

a. occipitofrontal
b. suboccipitobregmatic
c. bitemporal
d. biparietal

7–17. What is the approximate uteroplacental blood flow near term?

a. 100 to 200 mL/min
b. 300 to 450 mL/min

c. 700 to 900 mL/min
d. 1200 to 1400 mL/min

7–18. What is the estimated total surface area of the placenta at term?

a. 2 m^2
b. 10 m^2
c. 25 m^2
d. 55 m^2

7–19. What is the mechanism of transfer of anesthetic gases across the placenta?

a. simple diffusion
b. facilitated diffusion
c. active transport
d. pinocytosis

7–20. What is the PO$_2$ (mm Hg) of intervillous space blood?

a. 10 to 20 mm Hg
b. 30 to 35 mm Hg
c. 65 to 75 mm Hg
d. 90 to 95 mm Hg

7–21. What is the average oxygen saturation of intervillous space blood?

a. 10 to 15 percent
b. 25 to 35 percent
c. 65 to 75 percent
d. 90 to 95 percent

7–22. What is the average PO$_2$ (mm Hg) in the umbilical vein?

a. 15 mm Hg
b. 27 mm Hg
c. 49 mm Hg
d. 77 mm Hg

7–23. What is the average PO$_2$ (mm Hg) in the umbilical artery?

a. 15 mm Hg
b. 27 mm Hg
c. 49 mm Hg
d. 77 mm Hg

7–24. What is the mechanism of iron transport across the placenta?

a. active transfer
b. simple diffusion
c. facilitated diffusion
d. endocytosis

7–25. How is glucose transferred across the placenta?

    a. active transport
    b. simple diffusion
    c. facilitated diffusion
    d. endocytosis

7–26. How are amino acids transferred across the placenta?

    a. active transport
    b. simple diffusion
    c. facilitated diffusion
    d. endocytosis

7–27. Which of the following is an example of a large protein that readily crosses the placenta?

    a. IgG
    b. thyrotropin
    c. insulin
    d. IgM

7–28. How does IgG cross the placenta?

    a. active transport
    b. simple diffusion
    c. facilitated diffusion
    d. endocytosis

7–29. How do calcium and phosphorous cross the placenta?

    a. active transport
    b. simple diffusion
    c. facilitated diffusion
    d. endocytosis

7–30. Which of the following factors may play a significant role in fetal lung development?

    a. vitamin A
    b. cholecalciferol
    c. parathyroid–hormone-related protein
    d. epidermal growth factors

7–31. Which of the following fetal vessels empties directly into the inferior vena cava?

    a. umbilical
    b. portal
    c. ductus venosus
    d. hepatic

7–32. Which of the following contains the best oxygenated blood in the fetus?

    a. superior vena cava
    b. blood deflected by the crista dividens
    c. ductus arteriosus
    d. right ventricle

7–33. Which of the following structures represents the intra-abdominal remnants of the umbilical vein?

    a. umbilical ligaments
    b. ligamentum teres
    c. ligamentum venosus
    d. ligamentum portal

7–34. Which of the following fetal structures is NOT a site of early hematopoiesis?

    a. yolk sac
    b. liver
    c. bone marrow
    d. kidney

7–35. What is the approximate fetoplacental blood volume at term?

    a. 70 mL/kg
    b. 125 mL/kg
    c. 225 mL/kg
    d. 250 mL/kg

7–36. Which of the following hemoglobins contains a pair of alpha chains and a pair of gamma chains?

    a. Gower-1
    b. hemoglobin F
    c. hemoglobin A
    d. hemoglobin A_2

7–37. What percentage of total hemoglobin at birth is hemoglobin F?

    a. 5
    b. 38
    c. 75
    d. 99

7–38. Which of the following vitamins is important to be given prophylactically for the fetus soon after birth (especially in the breast-feeding newborn)?

    a. vitamin K
    b. vitamin A

c. vitamin C
d. vitamin D

7–39. The bulk of IgG acquired by the fetus from its mother occurs during which of the following time periods?

    a. 10 to 14 weeks
    b. 16 to 20 weeks
    c. 24 to 28 weeks
    d. last 4 weeks of pregnancy

7–40. Which of the following immunological factors provides protection against enteric infections when ingested in the colostrum?

    a. IgG
    b. IgM
    c. IgA
    d. IgE

7–41. At what gestational age will the fetus first demonstrate spontaneous movements if removed from the uterus?

    a. 8 weeks
    b. 10 weeks
    c. 12 weeks
    d. 14 weeks

7–42. How early might the fetus hear sounds in utero?

    a. 14th week
    b. 18th week
    c. 24th week
    d. 28th week

7–43. What is the average amount of amnionic fluid swallowed per 24 hours by the term fetus?

    a. 100 mL
    b. 200 mL
    c. 500 mL
    d. 1500 mL

7–44. At what gestational age is insulin first detectable in fetal plasma?

    a. 6 weeks
    b. 12 weeks
    c. 16 weeks
    d. 20 weeks

7–45. What is the approximate urine output per day of a term fetus?

    a. 100 mL
    b. 350 mL
    c. 650 mL
    d. 1000 mL

7–46. What is the approximate volume of amnionic fluid at 12 weeks' gestation?

    a. 10 mL
    b. 50 mL
    c. 150 mL
    d. 280 mL

7–47. Where is surfactant primarily produced in the fetal lung?

    a. type II pneumocytes
    b. alveoli macrophages
    c. alveoli basement membrane cells
    d. interstitial cells

7–48. Which of the following glycerophospholipids make up the vast majority of mature surfactant?

    a. phosphatidylinositol
    b. phosphatidylethanolamine
    c. phosphatidylglycerol
    d. phosphatidylcholine

7–49. Approximately what percentage of the glycerophospholipids of surfactant is made up of dipalmitoylphosphatidylcholine (lecithin)?

    a. 10
    b. 25
    c. 50
    d. 75

7–50. Which of the following compounds is the precursor of all glycerophospholipids of surfactant?

    a. inositol
    b. ethanolamine
    c. choline diphosphate
    d. phosphatidic acid

7–51. Which of the following is likely to be present at very low levels in the amnionic fluid of infants of diabetic mothers near term?

    a. dipalmitoylphosphatidylcholine
    b. phosphatidylinositol
    c. phosphatidylglycerol
    d. lecithin

7–52. What is the major surfactant-associated protein (apo-protein)?

    a. SP-A
    b. SP-B
    c. SP-C
    d. SP-D

7–53. Which of the following hormones, in concert with cortisol, is probably the lead hormone in the stimulation of surfactant biosynthesis in the fetal lung?

    a. prolactin
    b. estrogen
    c. progesterone
    d. thyroxine

7–54. When can movements of the fetal chest wall first be detected by ultrasound?

    a. 11 weeks
    b. 18 weeks
    c. 24 weeks
    d. 26 weeks

7–55. When can corticotropin first be detected in the fetal pituitary?

    a. 7 weeks
    b. 11 weeks
    c. 15 weeks
    d. 19 weeks

7–56. When does the fetal testis begin to secrete testosterone?

    a. 6 weeks
    b. 10 weeks
    c. 16 weeks
    d. 22 weeks

7–57. What is the most likely explanation for the 46,XX male?

    a. production of Müllerian-inhibiting substance by the ovary
    b. Y chromosome was lost from a 47,XXY fetus
    c. translocation of portions of the Y chromosome to the X chromosome
    d. error in karyotyping

7–58. Which of the following statements is correct regarding Müllerian-inhibiting substance?

    a. It is a hormone.
    b. It is produced by the Leydig cells.
    c. It acts locally near its site of formation.
    d. It appears after testosterone.

7–59. Which of the following is NOT characteristic of female pseudohermaphroditism?

    a. Müllerian-inhibiting substance is not produced.
    b. The fetus is exposed to androgen.
    c. The karyotype is 46,XX.
    d. A testis is present on one side.

7–60. Which of the following is NOT characteristic of male pseudohermaphroditism?

    a. Müllerian-inhibiting substance is produced.
    b. Androgenic representation is variable.
    c. Karyotype is 47,XXY.
    d. Testes or no gonads are present.

7–61. Which of the following is NOT characteristic of testicular feminization?

    a. female phenotype
    b. short, blind-ending vagina
    c. no uterus or fallopian tubes
    d. ovarian remnants on one side

8

Maternal Adaptations to Pregnancy

8–1. What is the average uterine weight at term?

    a. 200 g
    b. 450 g
    c. 780 g
    d. 1100 g

8–2. What is the approximate uteroplacental blood flow at term?

    a. 100 mL/min
    b. 250 mL/min
    c. 550 mL/min
    d. 800 mL/min

8–3. Which of the following is NOT a factor responsible for the changes seen in the cervix in early pregnancy

    a. decreased vascularity
    b. increased edema
    c. hypertrophy of cervical glands
    d. hyperplasia of cervical glands

8–4. Which of the following is NOT produced by the corpus luteum of early pregnancy?

    a. progesterone
    b. 17α-hydroxyprogesterone
    c. relaxin
    d. prolactin

8–5. Which of the following statements is NOT true regarding a luteoma of pregnancy?

    a. It is not a true neoplasm.
    b. It is a common cause of female fetal virilization.
    c. It may recur in subsequent pregnancies.
    d. It represents an exaggeration of luteinization.

8–6. How does hyperreactio luteinalis differ from a pregnancy luteoma?

    a. It is cystic compared with luteoma.
    b. It may cause maternal virilization.
    c. It has a different cellular pattern.
    d. It is associated with very low serum chorionic gonadotropin levels compared with the luteoma.

8–7. What is pigmentation of the midline of abdominal skin during pregnancy called?

    a. striae gravidarum
    b. linea nigra
    c. chloasma
    d. melasma

8–8. What is the average weight gain in the first trimester?

    a. 1 kg
    b. 5 kg
    c. 7 kg
    d. 9 kg

8–9. What is the average weight gain during pregnancy?

    a. 5 kg
    b. 9 kg
    c. 11 kg
    d. 15 kg

8–10. What is the minimum amount of extra water that the average woman retains during normal pregnancy?

    a. 1.0 L
    b. 3.5 L
    c. 6.5 L
    d. 8.0 L

8–11. Of the total 1000 g of protein increase induced by normal pregnancy, how much is utilized by the fetus and placenta?

    a. 100 g
    b. 300 g
    c. 500 g
    d. 750 g

8–12. Which one of the following does NOT contribute to beta cell hypertrophy, hyperplasia, and hypersecretion of insulin during pregnancy?

    a. human placental lactogen
    b. estrogen
    c. progesterone
    d. human chorionic gonadotropin

8–13. Which of the following statements is NOT true regarding carbohydrate metabolism during pregnancy?

    a. There is an increased insulin response to glucose.
    b. There is an increased peripheral uptake of glucose.
    c. There is a suppressed glucagon response.
    d. Increased concentrations of free fatty acids increase insulin resistance.

8–14. What causes the increase in HDL-cholesterol noted in the first half of pregnancy?

    a. prolactin
    b. estrogen
    c. progesterone
    d. hCG

8–15. What is responsible for the increase in LDL-cholesterol up to 36 weeks gestation?

    a. prolactin
    b. estrogen
    c. progesterone
    d. hCG

8–16. What is the average plasma bicarbonate level during pregnancy?

    a. 29 mmol/L
    b. 26 mmol/L
    c. 22 mmol/L
    d. 16 mmol/L

8–17. Which of the following statements best characterizes the acid–base status during pregnancy?

    a. There is a mild respiratory alkalosis.
    b. There is a mild respiratory acidosis.
    c. There is a mild metabolic alkalosis.
    d. There is a mild metabolic acidosis.

8–18. What is the average increase in maternal blood volume during pregnancy?

    a. 10%
    b. 25%
    c. 50%
    d. 75%

8–19. What is the average increase in the volume of circulating erythrocytes during pregnancy?

    a. 100 mL
    b. 250 mL
    c. 450 mL
    d. 700 mL

8–20. Which of the following hematologic changes does NOT occur during normal pregnancy?

    a. The mean age of circulating red cells is increased.
    b. The mean cell volume is increased.
    c. There is moderate erythroid hyperplasia.
    d. There is an increase in plasma erythropoietin.

8–21. Which of the following is NOT felt to be an effect of atrial natriuretic peptide?

    a. natriuresis
    b. diuresis
    c. increased basal release of aldosterone
    d. direct vasorelaxant action on vascular smooth muscle

8–22. What are the average iron stores of normal young women?

    a. 300 mg
    b. 500 mg
    c. 4 g
    d. 6 g

8–23. What are the iron requirements of normal pregnancy?

    a. 300 mg
    b. 500 mg

c. 1 g

d. 4 g

8–24. Approximately how much iron is required by the fetus during pregnancy?

a. 150 mg

b. 300 mg

c. 500 mg

d. 1 g

8–25. What are the average daily iron requirements during the second half of pregnancy?

a. 1 to 2 mg/day

b. 3.5 to 4.0 mg/day

c. 6 to 7 mg/day

d. 15 to 20 mg/day

8–26. Which of the following is NOT increased in pregnancy?

a. blood leukocyte count

b. C-reactive protein

c. leukocyte alkaline phosphate activity

d. α-interferon

8–27. What is the average increase in fibrinogen concentration during pregnancy?

a. 10%

b. 25%

c. 50%

d. 75%

8–28. Which of the following coagulation factors is NOT increased during pregnancy?

a. factor VII

b. factor VIII

c. factor IX

d. factor XI

8–29. What is the average increase in the resting pulse during pregnancy?

a. 0 to 1 bpm

b. 5 to 6 bpm

c. 10 to 15 bpm

d. 18 to 20 bpm

8–30. What is the average increase in cardiac volume between early and late pregnancy?

a. 75 mL

b. 150 mL

c. 250 mL

d. 350 mL

8–31. Which of the following is most likely responsible for the increase in the cardiac silhouette noted in radiographs in pregnant women?

a. displacement of the heart to the left and upward

b. cardiomegaly of pregnancy

c. increase in cardiac output

d. pericardial effusion of pregnancy

8–32. Which of the following changes in cardiac sounds is NOT found during pregnancy?

a. exaggerated splitting of the first heart sound

b. marked splitting of the aortic and pulmonary elements of the second sound

c. a systolic murmur in 90 percent of women

d. a diastolic murmur in 20 percent of women

8–33. What is the most characteristic electrocardiographic finding in normal pregnancy?

a. shortening of the QRS complex

b. shortening of the ST segment

c. slight depression of the ST segment

d. slight left axis deviation

8–34. In which of the following situations is cardiac output NOT increased?

a. left lateral recumbent position

b. first stage of labor

c. second stage of labor

d. supine position

8–35. Which of the following hemodynamic values remains unchanged during normal pregnancy?

a. systemic vascular resistance

b. pulmonary vascular resistance

c. colloid osmotic pressure

d. pulmonary capillary wedge pressure

8–36. Which of the following is NOT increased in normotensive pregnant women?

a. renin activity and renin concentration

b. angiotensin II

c. sensitivity to pressor effects of angiotensin II

d. aldosterone

8–37. Which of the following is least likely to be involved in the control of vascular reactivity during pregnancy?

 a. prostaglandins
 b. estrogens
 c. alteration in cyclic AMP
 d. changes in intracellular calcium concentrations

8–38. What is the average elevation of the diaphragm during normal pregnancy?

 a. 0 to 1 cm
 b. 2 cm
 c. 4 cm
 d. 6 cm

8–39. Which of the following is NOT increased in normal pregnancy?

 a. tidal volume
 b. minute ventilatory volume
 c. minute oxygen uptake
 d. functional residual capacity

8–40. Which of the following is NOT increased during normal pregnancy?

 a. glomerular filtration rate
 b. renal plasma flow
 c. creatinine clearance
 d. plasma concentration of urea

8–41. With regard to the hydronephrosis and hydroureter associated with pregnancy, which of the following is NOT true?

 a. Ureteral dilation is greater on the right side.
 b. Ureteral dilation is primarily due to hormonal factors.
 c. There is elongation of the ureters.
 d. There is increase in the number of curves of the ureters.

8–42. With regard to the liver during pregnancy, which of the following is MOST correct?

 a. Total alkaline phosphatase is decreased.
 b. Plasma albumin concentration is increased.
 c. Plasma cholinesterase activity is decreased.
 d. Leucine aminopeptidase activity is markedly decreased.

8–43. Which of the following statements is MOST correct regarding the pituitary gland during pregnancy?

 a. There is no change in the size of the pituitary gland.
 b. The maternal pituitary gland is not essential for maintenance of pregnancy.
 c. There is a marked increase in growth hormone.
 d. Prolactin increases only slightly in maternal plasma.

8–44. Which of the following shows the greatest increase in pregnancy?

 a. thyroxine-binding globulin (TBG).
 b. total thyroxine (T_4).
 c. total triiodothyronine (T_3).
 d. free thyroxine (T_4).

8–45. Which of the following is most likely to cross the placenta?

 a. thyroxine
 b. triiodothyronine
 c. reverse triiodothyronine
 d. thyroid-releasing hormone

8–46. Which of the following is NOT increased during pregnancy?

 a. parathyroid hormone
 b. serum calcium
 c. calcitonin
 d. size of the thyroid gland

8–47. Which of the following is NOT increased during normal pregnancy?

 a. serum concentration of circulating cortisol
 b. rate of cortisol secretion by the maternal adrenal
 c. maternal levels of deoxycorticosterone
 d. maternal levels of testosterone

8–48. At what rate is aldosterone secreted in the third trimester?

 a. 1 mg/day
 b. 2 mg/day
 c. 3 mg/day
 d. 4 mg/day

8–49. What is the level of testosterone in umbilical venous plasma likely to be in a pregnant woman with an androgen-secreting tumor?

    a. very high
    b. too low to be detected
    c. the same as in maternal serum
    d. none of the above

8–50. Which of the following increases during pregnancy?

    a. platelet concentration
    b. platelet size
    c. clotting time
    d. plasma fibrinogen level

8–51. What would be the expected result of deficient levels of antithrombin III, protein C, and protein S?

    a. extensive blood loss at delivery
    b. recurrent thromboembolic episodes
    c. recurrent abortion
    d. infertility

8–52. What is the purpose of the supine pressor test?

    a. predicts pregnancy-induced hypertension when an increase in 20 mmHg blood pressure is noted upon a change from lateral recumbent to the supine position
    b. may detect a placental abruption
    c. is useful in finding patients with Raynaud's disease
    d. is positive after smoking

Antepartum Management of Normal Pregnancy

| 9 |

Prenatal Care

9–1. What is the goal of prenatal care?

    a. to establish a good relationship with your patients

    b. to deliver a healthy baby without impairing the mother's health

    c. to set up a payment schedule for the delivery

    d. to see the patient often enough so you feel comfortable with the patient

9–2. By how much should fetal mortality be reduced due to organized prenatal care?

    a. 20%

    b. 40%

    c. 60%

    d. 80%

9–3. What is a primipara?

    a. a woman who was pregnant once

    b. a woman delivered once of a viable fetus

    c. a woman who has completed two pregnancies

    d. a woman who has had a 12-week miscarriage

9–4. What is a nulligravida?

    a. a woman who never delivered a live-born baby

    b. a woman who had one miscarriage

    c. a woman who has never been pregnant

    d. a woman who had only one pregnancy

9–5. What is the mean duration of pregnancy from the first day of the LMP?

    a. 250 days

    b. 260 days

    c. 270 days

    d. 280 days

9–6. Naegele's rule estimates gestation age based on which of the following formulas?

    a. Add 7 days to LMP and count back three months.

    b. Subtract 7 days from LMP and count back three months.

    c. Add 21 days to LMP and count back three months.

    d. Subtract 21 days from LMP and count back three months.

9–7. Which of the following should NOT be included at the first prenatal visit?

a. complete history and physical
b. obstetrical examination
c. hemoglobin A_{1c} determination
d. urinalysis for glucose, protein, and culture

9–8. Which of the following tests should be voluntary at the first prenatal visit?

a. serological test for syphilis
b. gonorrhea culture
c. urinalysis
d. human immunodeficiency virus

9–9. The presence of foamy, yellow liquid in the vagina is suggestive of which of the following?

a. normal vaginal secretions
b. Candida vaginitis
c. Trichomonas vaginalis
d. Chlamydia cervicitis

9–10. There is good correlation of fundal height in centimeters and gestational age during which weeks of gestation?

a. 14 to 32 weeks
b. 16 to 34 weeks
c. 18 to 32 weeks
d. 20 to 36 weeks

9–11. Which of the following is NOT a midpregnancy event that enhances the reliability of the estimated gestational age?

a. audible fetal heart tones with a stethoscope by 20 weeks
b. fundal height at umbilicus at 20 weeks
c. serum human chorionic gonadotropin level greater than 50,000 m/U
d. fetal movement by 20 to 21 weeks' gestation

9–12. At what gestational age should screening tests for gestational diabetes be performed?

a. at the first prenatal visit of women with a positive family history
b. between 20 and 24 weeks' gestation
c. between 24 and 28 weeks' gestation
d. between 32 and 36 weeks' gestation

9–13. What is the earliest gestational age audible fetal heart sounds will be present in 100 percent of live pregnancies?

a. 16 weeks
b. 18 weeks
c. 20 weeks
d. 22 weeks

9–14. What is the average total weight gain in healthy primigravidas?

a. 20.0 lb
b. 27.5 lb
c. 35.0 lb
d. 42.5 lb

9–15. What is the average weight gain from 20 weeks' gestation to term?

a. $\frac{1}{2}$ lb/week
b. 1 lb/week
c. $1\frac{1}{2}$ lb/week
d. 2 lbs/week

9–16. What is the maximum weight gain recommended by the National Academy of Sciences for underweight women?

a. 15 lb
b. 25 lb
c. 40 lb
d. 60 lb

9–17. Which nutrient during pregnancy is not adequately provided in diet alone?

a. calcium
b. magnesium
c. iron
d. folate

9–18. For pregnancy, the Food and Nutrition Board recommends a daily caloric increase of how much?

a. 100 Kcal
b. 300 Kcal
c. 500 Kcal
d. 1000 Kcal

9–19. What are the average daily iron requirements during the latter half of pregnancy?

a. 1 mg/day
b. 3 mg/day
c. 5 mg/day
d. 7 mg/day

9–20. To minimize the gastrointestinal side effects of iron, when is it recommended that patients take their iron?

   a. at bedtime
   b. with breakfast
   c. during the first trimester
   d. only if the hemoglobin is less than 10 mg/dL

9–21. What characterizes calcium absorption during pregnancy?

   a. decreases
   b. remains the same
   c. increases
   d. increases with vitamin E

9–22. During pregnancy, how much calcium is retained?

   a. 30 g
   b. 60 g
   c. 90 g
   d. 120 g

9–23. Which of the following is NOT associated with zinc deficiency?

   a. impaired wound healing
   b. poor appetite
   c. suboptimal growth
   d. diarrhea

9–24. What are the current recommendations for daily zinc intake?

   a. <1 mg
   b. 5 mg
   c. 15 mg
   d. 30 mg

9–25. What enzyme or compound is associated with copper?

   a. glutathione peroxidase
   b. glycosyltransferases
   c. cytochrome oxidase
   d. insulin

9–26. What cofactor for insulin facilitates the hormone's attachment to its peripheral receptors?

   a. selenium
   b. sodium
   c. manganese
   d. chromium

9–27. What enzyme or compound is associated with selenium?

   a. glutathione peroxidase
   b. glycosyltransferases
   c. cytochrome oxidase
   d. insulin

9–28. What enzyme or compound is associated with chromium?

   a. glutathione peroxidase
   b. glycosyltransferases
   c. cytochrome oxidase
   d. insulin

9–29. What enzyme or compound is associated with manganese?

   a. glutathione peroxidase
   b. glycosyltransferases
   c. cytochrome oxidase
   d. insulin

9–30. Which of the following is NOT associated with folate acid deficiency during pregnancy?

   a. hypersegmented neutrophils
   b. megaloblastic erythropoiesis
   c. increased infections
   d. megaloblastic anemia

9–31. Which of the following is recommended to prevent neural tube defects?

   a. vitamin A
   b. vitamin B6
   c. folate
   d. ascorbic acid

9–32. Excessive ingestion of which vitamin can lead to vitamin B_{12} deficiency?

   a. A
   b. B_6
   c. C
   d. D

9–33. What is the recommended daily dietary allowance for vitamin C during pregnancy?

   a. 10 mg
   b. 30 mg
   c. 50 mg
   d. 70 mg

9–34. What are the results of continuation of running and aerobic exercise programs during pregnancy?

    a. lower birthweight infants
    b. longer labors
    c. more midtrimester losses
    d. more fetal distress during labor

9–35. What are the hazards for pregnant women who work at jobs that require prolonged standing?

    a. delivering preterm
    b. fetal growth retardation
    c. preeclampsia
    d. preterm rupture of fetal membranes

9–36. What are the hazards of travel to the healthy pregnancy?

    a. decreased birthweight
    b. increased bleeding
    c. longer labors
    d. no risks identified

9–37. What are the risks of caffeine intake to the pregnancy?

    a. low birthweight
    b. increased anomalies
    c. increased mutagenesis
    d. none

9–38. What is the recommendation for the administration of hepatitis B vaccine to pregnant women?

    a. contraindicated
    b. same as for nonpregnant women
    c. for postexposure only
    d. only if risk factors are present

9–39. What is the recommendation for the administration of rabies vaccine to pregnant women?

    a. contraindicated
    b. same as for nonpregnant women
    c. for postexposure only
    d. only if risk factors are present

9–40. What is the recommendation for the administration of typhoid vaccine to pregnant women?

    a. contraindicated
    b. same as for nonpregnant women

    c. only if traveling to endemic area
    d. only if risk factors are present

9–41. What is the recommendation for the administration of plague vaccine to pregnant women?

    a. contraindicated
    b. same as for nonpregnant women
    c. for postexposure only
    d. only if traveling to endemic area

9–42. What is the recommendation for the administration of measles vaccine to pregnant women?

    a. contraindicated
    b. same as for nonpregnant women
    c. for postexposure only
    d. only if risk factors are present

9–43. What is the recommendation for the administration of pneumococcus vaccine to pregnant women?

    a. contraindicated
    b. same as for nonpregnant women
    c. for postexposure only
    d. only if risk factors are present

9–44. What is the recommendation for the administration of mumps vaccine to pregnant women?

    a. contraindicated
    b. same as for nonpregnant women
    c. for postexposure only
    d. only if risk factors are present

9–45. What is the proposed etiology for nausea and vomiting in the first trimester?

    a. increased human placenta lactogen
    b. increased chorionic gonadotropin
    c. decreased growth hormone
    d. decreased progesterone

9–46. Which of the following cravings does NOT signify severe iron deficiency anemia?

    a. ice
    b. dry lump starch
    c. clay
    d. iron

10

Lie, Presentation, Attitude, and Position of the Fetus

10–1. What is the relationship of the long axis of the fetus to that of the mother called?

   a. presentation of the fetus
   b. lie of the fetus
   c. fetal attitude
   d. fetal posture

10–2. What percentage of term labors present with a longitudinal lie?

   a. 50
   b. 75
   c. 90
   d. 99

10–3. What is the presentation when the fetal neck is extended and the back and occiput are in contact?

   a. vertex
   b. face
   c. brow
   d. sinciput

10–4. What is the presentation when the fetal head is flexed and the occipital fontanel is presenting?

   a. vertex
   b. face
   c. brow
   d. sinciput

10–5. What is the presentation when the fetal head is partially flexed and a large anterior fontanel is presenting?

   a. vertex
   b. face
   c. brow
   d. sinciput

10–6. What type of breech presents with the thighs flexed and legs extended?

   a. complete
   b. incomplete
   c. frank
   d. transverse lie

10–7. In shoulder presentations, what portion of the fetus is used to orient it with the maternal pelvis?

   a. humerus
   b. vertex
   c. acromion
   d. clavicle

10–8. In which of the following presentations does the fetal attitude (vertebral column) become concave (extended)?

   a. face
   b. shoulder
   c. cephalic
   d. breech

10–9. What is the incidence of breech presentation at 29 to 32 weeks' gestation?

   a. 7%
   b. 14%
   c. 21%
   d. 28%

10–10. What components make up the podalic pole?

   a. breech only
   b. extremities only
   c. breech and extremities
   d. none of the above

10–11. What Leopold maneuver involves grasping the lower portion of the abdomen just above the symphysis?

    a. 1st
    b. 2nd
    c. 3rd
    d. 4th

10–12. What Leopold maneuver involves fundal palpation to define the fetal pole present in the fundus?

    a. 1st
    b. 2nd
    c. 3rd
    d. 4th

10–13. What Leopold maneuver involves placing the palms of the hands on each side of the abdomen to determine the location of the back and small parts?

    a. 1st
    b. 2nd
    c. 3rd
    d. 4th

10–14. Which of the following maneuvers is NOT used in the vaginal examination to determine presentation and position?

    a. differentiate vertex from breech by digital examination
    b. sweep examining fingers posterior to anterior (i.e., across sagittal suture)
    c. determine position of the two fontanels
    d. determine position of the nose

10–15. With which of the following presentations will the fetal heart sounds be best heard a short distance from the midline?

    a. occipitoanterior
    b. occipitoposterior
    c. transverse
    d. breech

Normal Labor and Delivery

11

Parturition: Biomolecular and Physiologic Processes

11–1. Which of the following is essential for myometrial contractions?

    a. tubulin-actin
    b. actin-myosin
    c. myosin-tubulin
    d. all of the above

11–2. Which of the following is NOT true concerning smooth muscle contractions?

    a. The degree of shortening is greater than that of striated muscle.
    b. Force can be exerted in any direction.
    c. Muscle is arranged in long, random bundles.
    d. Expulsive force as a result of the contraction is unidirectional.

11–3. Which of the following is essential for the generation of smooth muscle contractions?

    a. prostaglandins
    b. intracellular free calcium

    c. extracellular free calcium
    d. oxytocin

11–4. Which of the following activates the phosphorylation reaction responsible for myometrial contractions?

    a. free intracellular calcium
    b. ATPase
    c. ATP hydrolysis
    d. myosin light chain kinase

11–5. Which of the following characterizes active labor?

	contraction duration (sec)	amniotic fluid pressure (mm)
a.	30	10
b.	30	20
c.	60	40
d.	90	80

11–6. What is the major site of estrogen formation during pregnancy?

    a. peripheral conversion
    b. ovary
    c. corpus luteum
    d. placenta

11–7. What is the direction of cervical effacement?

    a. outer edge inward
    b. above downward to outer edge
    c. midcervical canal bidirectional
    d. above downward with cervical fibers taken up into lower uterine segment

11–8. What is the most attractive hypothesis for the cause of labor pain?

    a. myometrial hypoxia
    b. cervical stretching
    c. peritoneum stretching
    d. compression of nerve ganglia in the cervix

11–9. What is the average amnionic fluid pressure generated by uterine contractions?

    a. 1 mm Hg
    b. 10 mm Hg
    c. 40 mm Hg
    d. 100 mm Hg

11–10. What causes the pathological Bandl ring?

    a. thinning of lower uterine segment
    b. thinning of upper uterus
    c. thickness of lower uterine segment
    d. a band of fibromuscular tissue at the level of the internal os

11–11. Which of the following is NOT a vital force concerned in labor?

    a. intra-abdominal pressure
    b. cervical position
    c. resistance
    d. uterine contractions

11–12. According to Friedman, what is the most important measure of labor progression?

    a. contraction frequency
    b. contraction intensity
    c. contraction duration
    d. cervical dilatation

11–13. During the preparatory division of labor, which of the following inhibits uterine contractions?

    a. sedation
    b. antibiotics
    c. bedrest
    d. warm baths

11–14. Which of the following is NOT a part of the urogenital diaphragm?

    a. sphincter ani
    b. deep perineal fascia
    c. middle perineal fascia
    d. superficial perineal fascia

11–15. Which of the following is NOT a muscle of the superficial perineal group?

    a. bulbocavernosus
    b. ischiocavernosus
    c. sphincter ani
    d. superficial transverse perineal muscle

11–16. Which protein may be important in the attachment of trophoblasts with the decidua?

    a. alphafetoprotein
    b. collagen type II
    c. oncofetal fibronectin
    d. transbinding globulin

11–17. In which of the following mammals are the events of parturition clearly established?

    a. man
    b. dolphin
    c. sheep
    d. horse

11–18. In most mammals the implementation of phase 1 of parturition is due to which of the following?

    a. cortisol withdrawal
    b. progesterone withdrawal
    c. increase in oxytocin receptors
    d. inflammatory responses (i.e., cytokines)

11–19. What is the fetal signal for commencement of parturition?

    a. withdrawal of progesterone
    b. deficient placenta estrogen
    c. increased fetal cortisol production
    d. no fetal signal

11–20. The increase in activity of which single enzyme causes progesterone withdrawal in sheep?

    a. 17-oxidoreductase
    b. 17 α-hydroxylase/17,20-lyase
    c. 3 β-hydroxysteroid dehydrogenase
    d. 17 β-hydroxylase

11–21. What actions are evoked by transforming growth factor-β?

    a. decrease prepro-endothelin-1 mRNA
    b. decrease immunoreactive PTH-γP protein secretion
    c. increase PTH-γP mRNA in myometrial cells
    d. fetal signal for parturition to start

11–22. What is an agent called that brings about the awakening of the uterus?

    a. contracting agent
    b. uterotropin
    c. uterotonin
    d. growth factor

11–23. Which of the following is not a uterotonin?

    a. endothelin-1
    b. prostaglandins
    c. oxytocin
    d. calcium

11–24. Which of the following characterizes phase 0 of parturition?

    a. myometrial tranquility
    b. uterine awakening
    c. cervical effacement
    d. cervical dilatation

11–25. Which of the following is NOT considered a structural component of the cervix?

    a. smooth muscle
    b. collagen
    c. ground substance
    d. oncofibronectin

11–26. At term, which of the following cervical components is decreased?

    a. hyaluronic acid
    b. dermatan sulfate
    c. collagen
    d. endocervical glands

11–27. What causes the increase in myometrial oxytocin receptors at term?

    a. increased oxytocin gene transcription
    b. increased oxytocin gene translation
    c. increased protein synthesis
    d. none of the above

11–28. Which of the following is NOT associated with phase 3 of parturition?

    a. uterine contractions
    b. milk ejection
    c. restoration of fertility
    d. uterine inversion

11–29. What is gap junction protein?

    a. actin
    b. myosin
    c. connexin
    d. laminin

11–30. Which of the following can block progesterone action?

    a. steroids
    b. RU-486
    c. aspirin
    d. β-blockers (i.e, inderal)

11–31. The human oxytocin receptor gene is located on which chromosome?

    a. 3
    b. 11
    c. 16
    d. X

11–32. What is one mechanism of oxytocin action?

    a. stimulate phosphatidylinositol hydrolysis
    b. decrease cyclic AMP
    c. stimulate prostaglandins
    d. decrease oxytocinase

11–33. What is the role of G-protein mediated activation of phospholipase C?

    a. blocks cAMP
    b. stimulates progesterone production
    c. activates arachidonic acid
    d. hydrolysis of phosphatidylinositol

11–34. What is the possible action of parathyroid hormone-related protein (PTH-γP)?

    a. vasorelaxant
    b. vasoconstrictor
    c. increases oxytocin receptors
    d. stimulates cervical ripening

11–35. Which of the following enzymes catalyzes the degradation of endothelin-1?

    a. endothelinase
    b. oxytocinase
    c. placental sulfatase
    d. enkephalinase

11–36. Where is oxytocin primarily synthesized?

    a. adrenal gland
    b. placenta
    c. posterior pituitary
    d. ovary

11–37. What is the carrier protein for oxytocin transport to the posterior pituitary?

    a. neurophysin
    b. relaxin
    c. binding globulin
    d. actin

11–38. Which of the following is an action of oxytocin?

    a. induces gap junction formation
    b. induces oxytocin receptors
    c. acts as an antiprogestin
    d. acts on amnion to facilitate amnionic fluid homeostasis

11–39. Which of the following is NOT evidence for a role of prostaglandins in human parturition?

    a. Prostaglandins will cause abortion at any stage of gestation
    b. Prostaglandins will cause labor at any stage of gestation.
    c. Levels of prostaglandins in the forebag are increased during labor.
    d. Prostaglandins cause contractions of smooth muscle cells in vitro.

11–40. Which of the following is a correct statement concerning arachidonic acid?

    a. There is a specific decrease in the AA content of phosphatidylinositol in the amnion early in labor.
    b. The maternal circulation provides AA for the fetus prior to 12 weeks.
    c. The AA content of amnion tissues increases during phase 2 of parturition.
    d. Later in the labor process the AA content is decreased.

11–41. What major prostaglandin is produced by the amnion?

    a. PGE_2
    b. PGF_2
    c. PGI
    d. PGG

11–42. What prostaglandin is preferentially produced by the decidua?

    a. PGE2
    b. $PGF_{2\alpha}$
    c. PGI
    d. PGG

11–43. What prostaglandin is produced by the chorion laeve in vitro?

    a. PGE2
    b. $PGF_{2\alpha}$
    c. PGG
    d. PGI

11–44. What is the initial and rate-limiting enzyme in prostaglandin inactivation?

    a. cyclooxygenase
    b. prostaglandin dehydrogenase
    c. enkephalinase
    d. oxytocinase

11–45. What percentage of pregnancies with suspected preterm labor remain undelivered without pharmacological intervention?

    a. 10
    b. 25
    c. 50
    d. 67

11–46. Which of the following is the action of platelet-activating factor (PAF) on myometrial cell?

    a. no effects on the myometrial cell
    b. decreases myosin light-chain kinase
    c. decreases Ca^{2+}
    d. increases Ca^{2+}

11–47. How does endothelin-1 increase the frequency of myometrial contractions in vitro?

    a. decreasing membrane-bound calcium
    b. decreasing total extracellular calcium
    c. increasing release of Ca^{2+} from membranes
    d. increasing release of Ca^{2+} from intracellular stores

11–48. What is the action of endothelin-1 on myometrial cells?

    a. decrease K^+ intracellular
    b. decrease Ca^{2+} intracellular
    c. increase K^+ intracellular
    d. increase Ca^{2+} intracellular

11–49. Which of the following tissues is avascularized?

    a. amnion
    b. syncytium
    c. decidua
    d. placenta

11–50. What is the incidence of preterm birth?

    a. 2%
    b. 4%
    c. 6%
    d. 12%

11–51. Which of the following bioactive agents is NOT a normal constituent of amnionic fluid?

    a. IL-1β
    b. IL-6
    c. MCSF
    d. prostaglandins

11–52. How often is interleukin-1β found in amnionic fluid of preterm pregnancies?

    a. 0
    b. 25%

    c. 33%
    d. 50%

11–53. What is the cell source of interleukin-1β in amnionic fluid?

    a. amnion
    b. chorion laeve
    c. cytotrophoblast
    d. mononuclear phagocytes

11–54. Which of the following cytokines stimulates the amnion cells to secrete IL-6 and IL-8?

    a. IL-1α
    b. IL-1β
    c. IL-4
    d. IL-12

11–55. Which of the following is a normal constituent of amnionic fluid?

    a. IL-1
    b. IL-2
    c. IL-4
    d. IL-8

11–56. What are the likely sources of the bioactive agent set in the amnionic fluid?

    a. chorion laeve; mononuclear cells
    b. chorion laeve; amnion
    c. decidual cells; mononuclear cells
    d. decidual cells; amnion

11–57. Which monumental event occurs during the second stage of labor?

    a. cervical effacement
    b. cervical dilatation
    c. expulsion of the fetus
    d. placenta separation

11–58. Which of the following is NOT a component of the paracrine arm of the fetal-maternal communication system?

    a. amnion
    b. chorion laeve
    c. decidua parietalis
    d. cytotrophoblasts

12

Mechanisms of Normal Labor in Occiput Presentation

12–1. What percentage of fetuses are in the occiput presentation at term?

    a. 80
    b. 85
    c. 90
    d. 95

12–2. What is the most common presentation of the fetus as it enters the pelvis?

    a. ROA
    b. ROT
    c. LOA
    d. LOT

12–3. What is the presentation if Leopold maneuvers reveal the following: (1) breech in fundus, (2) resistant plane palpated through mother's right flank, (3) head movable, (4) cephalic prominence on maternal left?

    a. ROT
    b. LOT
    c. LOA
    d. ROA

12–4. Posterior presentations are associated more commonly with which of the following?

    a. narrow forepelvis
    b. normal forepelvis
    c. wide forepelvis
    d. no association with forepelvis type

12–5. What are the cardinal movements of labor (in order)?

    a. descent, engagement, flexion, internal rotation, extension, external rotation, expulsion
    b. descent, flexion, engagement, internal rotation, extension, external rotation, expulsion
    c. engagement, descent, flexion, internal rotation, extension, external rotation, expulsion
    d. engagement, flexion, descent, internal rotation, extension, external rotation, expulsion

12–6. Which of the following is characteristic of asynclitism?

    a. Sagittal suture is not parallel to the transverse axis of the inlet.
    b. Sagittal suture lies midway between the symphysis and sacral promontory.
    c. Sagittal suture, although parallel to the transverse axis of the inlet, does not lie exactly midway between the symphysis and sacral promontory.
    d. Sagittal suture rotates 45 degrees from the sacral spines.

12–7. The chin is brought into intimate contact with the fetal thorax during which cardinal movement of labor?

    a. flexion
    b. extension
    c. engagement
    d. descent

12–8. The anterior shoulder appears under the symphysis during which cardinal movement of labor?

    a. extension
    b. expulsion
    c. external rotation
    d. descent

12–9. The biparietal diameter passes through the pelvic inlet during which cardinal movement of labor?

    a. descent
    b. engagement
    c. expulsion
    d. extension

12–10. During which cardinal movement of labor is the head returned to the oblique position?

    a. internal rotation
    b. extension
    c. external rotation
    d. expulsion

12–11. The base of the occiput is brought into contact with the inferior margin of the symphysis during which cardinal movement of labor?

    a. extension
    b. expulsion
    c. descent
    d. flexion

12–12. Which of the following is NOT one of the four forces of descent?

    a. pressure of amnionic fluid
    b. direct fundal pressure on the breech
    c. myometrial contractions
    d. contraction of abdominal muscles

12–13. During labor in the occiput posterior position, the occiput has to rotate to the symphysis pubis how many degrees?

    a. 45
    b. 90
    c. 135
    d. 180

12–14. What is edematous swelling of the fetal scalp during labor?

    a. molding
    b. caput succedaneum
    c. subdural hematoma
    d. erythema nodusum

12–15. Which of the following bones is most likely pushed under the parietal bones during molding?

    a. frontal
    b. the ipsilateral parietal bone
    c. temporal
    d. occipital

13

Conduct of Normal Labor and Delivery

13–1. Which of the following is characteristic of true labor?

a. irregular contractions
b. discomfort in lower abdomen
c. cervical dilatation
d. discomfort relieved by sedation

13–2. When should the fetal heart rate be auscultated during observation for labor?

a. before the contraction
b. during the contraction
c. at the end and immediately after a contraction
d. anytime

13–3. What is the station where the presenting part is at the level of the ischial spines?

a. −2
b. −1
c. 0
d. +1

13–4. What is the station where the fetal head is visible at the introitus?

a. +2
b. +3
c. +4
d. +5

13–5. What is the most reliable indicator of rupture of the fetal membranes?

a. fluid per cervical os
b. positive nitrazine test
c. positive ferning
d. positive oncofetal fibronectin

13–6. The nitrazine test for rupture of membranes may be false-positive if which of the following is present?

a. candida
b. vaginal bleeding
c. cervical mucus
d. bacterial vaginosis

13–7. What is the average duration of the first stage of labor in nulliparous women?

a. 5 hr
b. 8 hr
c. 12 hr
d. 20 hr

13–8. How often during the first stage of labor should the fetal heart rate be auscultated in a low-risk pregnancy?

a. every 15 min before a contraction
b. every 15 min after a contraction
c. every 30 min before a contraction
d. every 30 min after a contraction

13–9. How often during the first stage of labor should the fetal heart rate be auscultated in a high-risk pregnancy?

a. every 15 min before a contraction
b. every 15 min after a contraction
c. every 30 min before a contraction
d. every 30 min after a contraction

13–10. How often should the fetal heart rate be auscultated during the second stage of labor in low- versus high-risk patients?

a. 5 min/5 min
b. 10 min/5 min

c. 15 min/5 min

d. 30 min/5 min

13–11. Which of the following is noted when universal electronic fetal monitoring is compared to selective monitoring?

    a. increase in cesarean sections for fetal distress

    b. decrease in intrapartum deaths

    c. decrease in neonatal deaths

    d. decrease in low Apgar scores at 5 minutes

13–12. What is the median duration of the second stage of labor in multiparas?

    a. 5 min

    b. 10 min

    c. 20 min

    d. 30 min

13–13. What is the median duration of the second stage of labor in primiparas?

    a. 5 min

    b. 20 min

    c. 50 min

    d. 100 min

13–14. Which of the following is associated with a shortened second stage of labor?

    a. standing position

    b. squatting position

    c. supine position

    d. left lateral position

13–15. What is the encirclement of the largest diameter of the fetal head by the vulvar ring called?

    a. Bandl's ring

    b. crowning

    c. complete dilatation or beginning of second stage

    d. beginning of third stage of labor

13–16. What percentage of deliveries are complicated by a nuchal cord?

    a. 1

    b. 5

    c. 10

    d. 25

13–17. During the third stage of labor, which of the following is NOT a sign of placenta separation?

    a. a gush of blood

    b. uterus rises in the abdomen

    c. umbilical cord protrudes out of the vagina

    d. a sudden, sharp, unrelenting contraction

13–18. Which of the following is a complication of the third stage of labor associated with forced placental separation?

    a. endometritis

    b. uterine atony

    c. Asherman syndrome

    d. uterine inversion

13–19. What is the primary mechanism of placental site hemostasis?

    a. vasoconstriction by contracted myometrium

    b. oxytocin

    c. ergonovine maleate

    d. methylergonovine

13–20. What is the half-life of oxytocin?

    a. <1 min

    b. 3 to 5 min

    c. 10 to 15 min

    d. 20 to 30 min

13–21. Which deleterious effect is associated with oxytocin when given intravenously as a 10-unit bolus?

    a. hypertension

    b. hypotension

    c. oliguria

    d. polyuria

13–22. At what dosage of oxytocin should you expect to see a decrease in uterine blood flow?

    a. 10 μm/min

    b. 20 μm/min

    c. 30 μm/min

    d. 40 μm/min

13–23. How long does it take the antidiuretic effect of parenteral oxytocin to disappear after the infusion is stopped?

    a. <10 min
    b. 30 min
    c. 60 min
    d. 120 min

13–24. Which of thep6.5 following is associated with ergonovine and methylergonovine?

    a. seizures
    b. hypertension
    c. oliguria
    d. thrombocytopenia

13–25. What is a laceration involving the skin, mucous membrane, perineal body, anal sphincter, and rectal mucosa called?

    a. 1st degree
    b. 2nd degree
    c. 3rd degree
    d. 4th degree

13–26. What is a laceration involving the fourchette or perineal skin, but not the muscle, called?

    a. 1st degree
    b. 2nd degree
    c. 3rd degree
    d. 4th degree

13–27. What is a laceration involving the skin, mucous membrane, perineal body, and anal sphincter called?

    a. 1st degree
    b. 2nd degree
    c. 3rd degree
    d. 4th degree

13–28. What is the major advantage of a mediolateral episiotomy?

    a. easy surgical repair
    b. less postoperative pain
    c. less blood loss
    d. less extensions

13–29. Which factors are associated with an increased risk of third degree laceration?

    a. nulliparity, second-stage labor arrest, local anesthetics
    b. multiparity, second-stage labor arrest, local anesthetics
    c. nulliparity, precipitous second stage of labor, local anesthetics
    d. multiparity, precipitous second stage of labor, local anesthetics

13–30. Which of the following is not a morbidity associated with fourth degree lacerations?

    a. dehiscences
    b. infections
    c. uterine atony
    d. pain

14

Intrapartum Assessment

14–1. Which of the following is NOT linked to an abnormal fetal heart rate pattern?

    a. low 5-min Apgar
    b. fetal death
    c. neonatal death
    d. abnormal neurological outcomes

14–2. What portion of the fetal electrocardiogram is most reliably detected?

    a. p wave
    b. QRS complex
    c. R wave peak
    d. T wave

14–3. During electronic fetal monitoring how is a premature atrial contraction recorded?

    a. pause
    b. acceleration
    c. deceleration
    d. not detected

14–4. What is the purpose of attaching the reference electrode to the maternal thigh?

    a. serves as a ground
    b. eliminates electrical interference
    c. to differentiate between fetal and maternal signal
    d. to record maternal temperature

14–5. What term indicates that fetal heart rate has regularity whereas noise is random?

    a. autoregulation
    b. automation
    c. autocorrelation
    d. randomization

14–6. What are the usual settings for vertical and horizontal scaling during electronic monitoring?

    a. 30 bpm; 1 cm/min
    b. 30 bpm; 3 cm/min
    c. 60 bpm; 1 cm/min
    d. 60 bpm; 3 cm/min

14–7. Which of the following is responsible for the baseline fetal heart rate decreasing from 16 weeks to term?

    a. sympathetic response
    b. parasympathetic response
    c. increasing size of fetus
    d. hormonal alterations

14–8. What is the normal average baseline fetal heart rate at term?

    a. 100 to 140 bpm
    b. 110 to 150 bpm
    c. 120 to 160 bpm
    d. 120 to 140 bpm

14–9. What is bradycardia?

    a. baseline fetal heart rate < 100 for > 5 min
    b. baseline fetal heart rate < 100 for > 15 min

    c. baseline fetal heart rate < 120 for > 5 min
    d. baseline fetal heart rate < 120 for > 15 min

14–10. Which of the following is NOT associated with fetal bradycardia?

    a. head compression
    b. congenital heart block
    c. fetal compromise
    d. aminophylline

14–11. Which of the following defines severe bradycardia?

    a. <60 bpm for 1 min
    b. <80 bpm for 1 min
    c. <60 bpm for 3 min
    d. <80 bpm for 3 min

14–12. What is severe tachycardia?

    a. 161 bpm
    b. 181 bpm
    c. 201 bpm
    d. 221 bpm

14–13. What is the most common cause of fetal tachycardia?

    a. drug-induced
    b. maternal fever
    c. thyroid storm
    d. cardiac arrhythmias

14–14. What is the single most reliable sign of fetal compromise?

    a. fetal bradycardia
    b. fetal tachycardia
    c. reduced baseline variability
    d. repetitive severe variable decelerations

14–15. Which of the following is characteristic of sinusoidal fetal heart rate patterns?

    a. stable baseline with oscillation of 6 cycles/min
    b. stable baseline; amplitude of 5 to 15 bpm; and 2 to 5 cycles/min long-term variability
    c. unstable baseline with oscillation of 6 cycles/min
    d. unstable baseline; amplitude of 5 to 15 bpm and 2 to 5 cycles/min long-term variability

14–16. What is the frequency of sine waves when due to fetal anemia?

    a. 1 cycle/min
    b. 3 cycles/min
    c. 6 cycles/min
    d. 12 cycles/min

14–17. How are accelerations defined?

    a. increase in fetal heart rate of 10 bpm for 10 sec
    b. increase in fetal heart rate of 15 bpm for 10 sec
    c. increase in fetal heart rate of 10 bpm for 15 sec
    d. increase in fetal heart rate of 15 bpm for 15 sec

14–18. What is a drop in the fetal heart rate associated with the uterine contraction called?

    a. early deceleration
    b. late deceleration
    c. variable deceleration
    d. acceleration

14–19. What is a gradual, smooth descent of the fetal heart rate 30 sec after the contraction called?

    a. early deceleration
    b. late deceleration
    c. variable deceleration
    d. acceleration

14–20. What is the most common deceleration pattern encountered during labor?

    a. late decelerations
    b. early decelerations
    c. variable decelerations
    d. mixed decelerations

14–21. What is the cause of variable decelerations?

    a. head compression
    b. acidemia
    c. cord compression
    d. hypoxia

14–22. What are significant variable decelerations?

    a. fetal heart rate < 90 bpm for > 30 sec
    b. fetal heart rate < 70 bpm for > 30 sec
    c. fetal heart rate < 90 bpm for > 60 sec
    d. fetal heart rate < 70 bpm for > 60 sec

14–23. Which fetal heart rate pattern is NOT associated with an increase in fetal compromise?

    a. abnormal baseline rate less than 120
    b. absent beat-to-beat variability
    c. abnormal baseline rate more than 160
    d. repetitive mild variable decelerations

14–24. For which of the following is amnioinfusion not employed?

    a. meconium
    b. amniotic fluid index less than 3
    c. chorioamnionitis
    d. variable decelerations during labor

14–25. Which of the following represents a unique fetal heart-rate tracing characteristic of impaired neurological development as described by Shields and Schifrin?

    a. prolonged bradycardia (<100 bpm) for 30 minutes
    b. normal baseline rate with absent variability, mild variables with overshoot
    c. absent beat-to-beat variability with occasional late decelerations
    d. severe late decelerations with good beat-to-beat variability

14–26. What is the definition of asphyxia?

    a. fetal distress
    b. hypoxia leading to acidemia
    c. acidemia alone
    d. severe variable decelerations

14–27. What are the effects of using electronic fetal monitoring?

    a. improved perinatal outcome
    b. increased incidence of forceps delivery
    c. increased incidence of primary cesarean sections
    d. improved the care of the mother during labor

14–28. What are the current recommendations for auscultation of fetal heart rate in high risk pregnancies?

    a. first stage labor every 30 min; second stage every 15 min
    b. first stage labor every 30 min; second stage every 5 min

c. first stage labor every 15 min; second stage every 15 min

d. first stage labor every 15 min; second stage every 5 min

14–29. How is a Montevideo unit defined?

a. an increased pressure above baseline multiplied by the contraction frequency in 10 min

b. the number of contractions in 1 hr times the peak contraction pressure

c. the minimum contraction frequency in 10 min times the average contraction pressure

d. the number of contractions in 10 min times the amount of pitocin infused per hour

14–30. At what intensity are uterine contractions clinically palpable?

a. 5 mm Hg

b. 10 mm Hg

c. 20 mm Hg

d. 30 mm Hg

14–31. In humans, at what speed does the contraction spread from the pacemaker area throughout the uterus?

a. 0.5 cm/sec

b. 1.0 cm/sec

c. 2.0 cm/sec

d. 4.0 cm/sec

14–32. Before one decides to perform a cesarean section for dystocia, there should be how much uterine activity?

a. 75 to 100 Montevideo units

b. 150 to 175 Montevideo units

c. 200 to 225 Montevideo units

d. 300 to 325 Montevideo units

15

Analgesia and Anesthesia

15–1. What percentage of direct maternal deaths are secondary to anesthesia complications?

a. <1

b. 3 to 4

c. 6 to 8

d. 12 to 16

15–2. Which maternal finding is NOT an anesthesia risk factor?

a. anatomic anomaly of the face

b. asthma

c. morbid obesity

d. mild hypertension

15–3. Which of the following is a prominent cause of placental hypoperfusion?

a. hypotonic uterine contractions

b. severe preeclampsia

c. placenta previa

d. hyperthyroidism

15–4. Which of the following characterizes women who received continuous emotional support during labor?

a. deliver by cesarean section

b. request epidural analgesia

c. need oxytocin during labor

d. have less pain

15–5. When does the peak analgesia effect of meperidine given intramuscularly occur?

    a. <5 min
    b. 20 min
    c. 45 min
    d. 60 min

15–6. When does the peak analgesia effect of meperidine given intravenously occur?

    a. <5 min
    b. 20 min
    c. 45 min
    d. 60 min

15–7. Butorphanol administration has been associated with which fetal heart rate abnormality?

    a. repetitive late decelerations
    b. fetal tachycardia
    c. sinusoidal rhythm
    d. saltatory patter

15–8. What dose of butorphanol is comparable to 50 mg of meperidine?

    a. 0.5 mg IV
    b. 1 to 2 mg IV
    c. 4 to 5 mg IV
    d. 10 mg IV

15–9. What is the mechanism of action of naloxone hydrochloride?

    a. stimulates acetylcholinesterase
    b. displaces narcotic from specific receptors
    c. inhibits muscarinic receptors
    d. blocks beta receptors

15–10. Which physiological event causes the concentration of inhalation anesthetic to increase more rapidly in a pregnant women's lungs?

    a. increased tidal volume
    b. decreased functional residual capacity
    c. increased residual volume
    d. decreased total lung capacity

15–11. Which of the following is an occasional side effect of halothane anesthesia?

    a. anemia
    b. thrombocytopenia
    c. hypertension
    d. hepatitis

15–12. Which of the following is NOT associated with general anesthesia?

    a. decreased blood loss at cesarean section
    b. neonatal depression
    c. a significantly increased risk of early pregnancy loss in operating room personnel
    d. prolonged hospitalization

15–13. What is the advantage of ketamine when compared to thiopental?

    a. is not associated with hypotension
    b. causes delirium
    c. causes hallucinations
    d. induces general anesthesia at very low doses (<0.5 mg/kg)

15–14. What is one of the most common causes of anesthetic death in obstetrics?

    a. failed intubation
    b. hemorrhage
    c. pneumonitis
    d. stroke

15–15. Which of the following antacids has been associated with aspiration pneumonitis?

    a. bicitrate
    b. milk of magnesia
    c. cimetidine
    d. ranitidine

15–16. What is pressure on the cricoid cartilage (to occlude esophagus) called?

    a. Heimlich maneuver
    b. Circus maneuver
    c. Serrick maneuver
    d. Hawaiian maneuver

15–17. What amount of time is required after IV administered cimetidine to decrease gastric acidity?

    a. 15 min
    b. 60 min
    c. 2 hr
    d. 4 hr

15–18. Chemical pneumonitis develops if the gastric pH that is aspirated is less than which of the following?

   a. 2.5
   b. 3.0
   c. 4.0
   d. 5.0

15–19. What are the signs of aspiration of acidic liquid?

   a. bradycardia, decreased respirations, hypotension
   b. bradycardia, increased respirations, hypertension
   c. tachycardia, decreased respirations, hypotension
   d. tachycardia, increased respirations, hypotension

15–20. Which nerve roots are responsible for early first-stage labor pain?

   a. T_{10}, T_{11}
   b. T_{11}, T_{12}
   c. T_{10}, T_{11}, T_{12}, L_1
   d. S_2, S_3, S_4

15–21. Which nerve roots are responsible for late first-stage labor pain?

   a. T_{10}, T_{11}
   b. T_{11}, T_{12}
   c. T_{10}, T_{11}, T_{12}, L_1
   d. S_2, S_3, S_4

15–22. Which of the following is NOT a sign of central nervous system (CNS) toxicity from local anesthetics?

   a. slurred speech
   b. tinnitus
   c. paresthesia (mouth)
   d. hypertension

15–23. Which central acting agent is used to control convulsions caused by anesthetic-induced CNS toxicity?

   a. succinylcholine
   b. thiopental
   c. magnesium sulfate
   d. phenytoin

15–24. Which of the following is generally true concerning cardiovascular manifestations from local anesthetic toxicity?

   a. develop before CNS toxicity
   b. develop with CNS toxicity
   c. develop later than CNS toxicity
   d. no cardiovascular manifestations from local anesthetic toxicity

15–25. What is the most common complication of paracervical block?

   a. maternal hypotension
   b. CNS toxicity
   c. fetal bradycardia
   d. bleeding

15–26. What is the etiology of spinal headaches?

   a. puncture of meninges followed by leaking fluid
   b. hypotension after spinal block
   c. vasodilation of cerebral vessels
   d. drug-induced hormonal changes

15–27. Which of the following are absolute contraindications to spinal analgesia?

   a. preeclampsia
   b. infected skin at site of needle entry
   c. convulsions secondary to seizure disorders
   d. diabetes

15–28. Which of the following nerve blocks would provide complete analgesia for labor pain and vaginal delivery?

   a. T_8-S_2
   b. T_{10}-S_5
   c. T_{12}-S_2
   d. T_8-L_4

15–29. What is the most common side effect of epidural anesthesia?

   a. maternal hypertension
   b. maternal hypotension
   c. CNS stimulation
   d. ineffective block

15–30. What is the major advantage to using combination opiate and local anesthetic for epidural blockade?

    a. longer anesthesia effect
    b. less toxicity
    c. more rapid onset of pain relief
    d. increase in shivering

15–31. Which of the following local anesthetics has a rapid onset of action?

    a. chloroprocaine
    b. tetracaine
    c. lidocaine
    d. bupivicaine

16

The Newborn Infant

16–1. Which of the following characterizes fetal breathing?

    a. regular breathing
    b. episodic breathing
    c. deep inhalations
    d. long expirations

16–2. Which of the following contributes to transient tachypnea of the newborn?

    a. delay in removal of fluid from alveoli
    b. hypoxia
    c. hypercapnea
    d. hypothermia

16–3. Which of the following stimulates newborn respiration?

    a. O_2 accumulation and CO_2 accumulation
    b. O_2 accumulation and CO_2 deprivation
    c. O_2 deprivation and CO_2 deprivation
    d. O_2 deprivation and CO_2 accumulation

16–4. What Apgar score would you assign to a male infant at 5 minutes of life whose respiratory effort is irregular, pulse is 90, who is floppy and blue and with only minimal grimaces?

    a. 1
    b. 3
    c. 5
    d. 7

16–5. What is the significance of the 1-minute Apgar score?

    a. represents infant who needs special attention
    b. represents infant with birth asphyxia
    c. represents infant doomed to neurologic compromise
    d. represents infant that is normal

16–6. Which of the following is NOT part of the Apgar score?

    a. heart rate
    b. respiratory effort
    c. color
    d. amniotic fluid consistency

16–7. What is the risk of cerebral palsy in an infant with a 5-minute Apgar score less than or equal to 3?

    a. no increased risk over general population
    b. 1%
    c. 3%
    d. 10%

16–8. What percentage of children with cerebral palsy had normal Apgar scores?

    a. 10
    b. 25
    c. 50
    d. 75

16–9. Which of the following is NOT a criteria for intrapartum hypoxia associated with cerebral palsy?

  a. Apgar < 3 cm at 10 min
  b. seizures
  c. hypotonia
  d. respiratory acidemia

16–10. Which of the following neurologic deficits is related to perinatal asphyxia?

  a. mental retardation
  b. epilepsy
  c. hypotonia
  d. cerebral palsy

16–11. What is the definition of acidemia?

  a. decreased hydrogen ion concentration in umbilical artery blood
  b. increased hydrogen ion concentration in umbilical artery blood
  c. decreased oxygen concentration in umbilical artery blood
  d. increased oxygen concentration in umbilical artery blood

16–12 Which pH is considered clinically significant for fetal acidemia?

  a. pH < 7.20
  b. pH < 7.15
  c. pH < 7.10
  d. pH < 7.0

16–13. Which umbilical artery blood gas represents the mean expected in a normal-term infant?

  a. pH 7.35 pCO_2 49 mm Hg HCO_3 10 mEq/L
  b. pH 7.35 pCO_2 38 mm Hg HCO_3 23 mEq/L
  c. pH 7.28 pCO_2 49 mm Hg HCO_3 10 mEq/L
  d. pH 7.28 pCO_2 38 mm Hg HCO_3 23 mEq/L

16–14. Which of the following represents the mean umbilical vein blood gas analysis in a normal-term infant?

  a. pH 7.35 pCO_2 49 mm Hg HCO_3 10 mEq/L
  b. pH 7.35 pCO_2 38 mm Hg HCO_3 21 mEq/L
  c. pH 7.28 pCO_2 49 mm Hg HCO_3 10 mEq/L
  d. pH 7.28 pCO_2 38 mm Hg HCO_3 21 mEq/L

16–15. A blood gas analysis result of Ua pH 7.1; pCO_2 65 mm Hg; HCO_3 24 corresponds to which acidosis type?

  a. metabolic
  b. mixed
  c. respiratory
  d. normal

16–16. A blood gas analysis result of Ua pH 7.1; pCO_2 65 mm Hg; HCO_3 14 corresponds to which acidosis type?

  a. metabolic
  b. mixed
  c. respiratory
  d. normal

16–17. A blood gas analysis result of Ua pH 7.1; pCO_2 58 mm Hg; HCO_3 10 corresponds to which acidosis type?

  a. metabolic
  b. mixed
  c. respiratory
  d. normal

16–18. Which of the following is NOT a criterion to establish hypoxia near delivery as a cause of hypoxic ischemic encephalopathy?

  a. Ua pH < 7.00
  b. Apgar < 3
  c. hypertonia
  d. multiorgan system failure

16–19. Which of the following is NOT part of neonatal resuscitation?

  a. percentage of heat loss
  b. open airway
  c. positive pressure ventilation if needed
  d. oxygen for peripheral cyanosis

16–20. What is the pressure needed to effectively deliver O_2 via a face mask to a newborn?

   a. 1 cm H_2O
   b. 10 cm H_2O
   c. 20 cm H_2O
   d. 50 cm H_2O

16–21. What is the pressure required to effectively deliver O_2 via an endotracheal tube to a newborn?

   a. <1 cm H_2O
   b. 1 to 5 cm H_2O
   c. 10 to 20 cm H_2O
   d. 25 to 35 cm H_2O

16–22. Which of the following is a truly effective prophylaxis against chlamydial conjunctivitis in the newborn?

   a. 1% silver nitrate
   b. 2.5% povidone-iodine solution
   c. 0.5% erythromycin ointment
   d. none of the above

16–23. Which of the following will NOT be prevented by circumcision?

   a. phimosis
   b. epiphimosis
   c. paraphimosis
   d. balanoposthitis

Abnormal Labor

17

Dystocia: Abnormalities of Expulsive Forces

17–1. What is the most common cause of dystocia?

    a. pelvic contraction
    b. uterine dysfunction
    c. faulty presentation
    d. pelvic contractions and uterine dysfunction

17–2. What is the most common cause of primary cesarean section?

    a. malpresentation
    b. placental abruption
    c. prematurity
    d. dystocia

17–3. According to Friedman, what are the phases of cervical dilatation?

    a. preparatory-active
    b. preparatory-latent
    c. active-latent
    d. active pelvic

17–4. According to Friedman, what is prolongation of the latent phase of labor in a primigravida?

    a. 14 hr
    b. 20 hr
    c. 24 hr
    d. 48 hr

17–5. In the parous woman, how is the prolonged latent phase defined?

    a. >6 hr
    b. >14 hr
    c. >20 hr
    d. >24 hr

17–6. Which factor likely contributes to the prolongation of the latent phase?

    a. excessive sedation
    b. conduction analgesia
    c. uneffaced and undilated cervix
    d. all of the above

17–7. In a primigravida, what is the minimum rate of dilation of the cervix in the active phase of labor?

    a. 0.5 cm/hr
    b. 1.2 cm/hr
    c. 1.5 cm/hr
    d. 2.0 cm/hr

17–8. What is labor?

    a. painless, regular uterine contractions
    b. progressive cervical dilatation and effacement
    c. painful contractions every 2 to 3 minutes
    d. three contractions per 10 minutes

17–9. Which of the following is characteristic of the preparatory division of labor?

    a. change in cervical ground substance
    b. irregular contractions
    c. marked cervical dilatation
    d. rupture of membranes

17–10. According to Rosen, the active phase of labor begins at what dilatation?

    a. 3 cm
    b. 4 cm
    c. 5 cm
    d. 3 cm, if completely effaced

17–11. What is the mean duration of active-phase labor in nulliparous women?

    a. <3 hr
    b. 4 to 5 hr
    c. 6 to 8 hr
    d. ~12 hr

17–12. What is the median duration of second-stage labor in nulliparas and multiparas, respectively?

    a. 2 hr, 1 hr
    b. 2 hr, 30 min
    c. 50 min, 50 min
    d. 50 min, 20 min

17–13. Where in the myometrium do uterine contractions of normal labor begin and last longest?

    a. fundus
    b. lower uterine segment
    c. cervix
    d. laterally in miduterus

17–14. What amplitude of a uterine contraction is generally necessary to effect cervical dilatation?

    a. 5 mm Hg
    b. 15 mm Hg

    c. 25 mm Hg
    d. 50 mm Hg

17–15. Ninety-five percent of women admitted to a hospital in active labor will deliver spontaneously within how many hours?

    a. 4 hr
    b. 6 hr
    c. 10 hr
    d. 14 hr

17–16. In a multiparous woman, secondary arrest of dilatation is defined as no cervical dilatation for how long?

    a. >1 hr
    b. >2 hr
    c. >3 hr
    d. >14 hr

17–17. What is the preferred treatment for a nulliparous patient with prolonged deceleration phase and no signs of cephalopelvic disproportion?

    a. sedation
    b. oxytocin
    c. cesarean section
    d. increased hydration

17–18. Which of the following is NOT associated with a prolonged second stage of labor?

    a. congenital anomalies
    b. infant mortality
    c. infection
    d. postpartum hemorrhage

17–19. Which prostaglandin has been used for cervical ripening?

    a. $F_{2\alpha}$
    b. E_2
    c. $F_{2\beta}$
    d. E_1

17–20. What is the mean half-life of oxytocin in plasma?

    a. 5 min
    b. 10 min
    c. 15 min
    d. 20 min

17–21. How long does it take oxytocin to reach steady state levels in the plasma?

   a. 5 min
   b. 10 min
   c. 20 min
   d. 40 min

17–22. Which of the following is NOT true of hypertonic dysfunction?

   a. may be associated with placental abruption
   b. painful contraction
   c. ineffective cervical dilation
   d. occurs usually after 4 cm

17–23. Which of the following is true in a patient near term with rupture of membranes not in labor?

   a. Induction is mandatory.
   b. Within 24 hours 75 percent will enter labor spontaneously.
   c. Culture for group B strep is necessary.
   d. Early induction is associated with a decrease in the cesarean section rate.

17–24. How are Montevideo units are calculated?

   a. number of contractions in 10 min × peak amplitude
   b. number of contractions in 20 min × peak amplitude
   c. number of contractions in 30 min × peak amplitude
   d. add the peak amplitude minus the baseline for each contraction in a 10-min period

17–25. A patient with a missed abortion receives oxytocin at 60 mU per minute using D_5W for 14 hours. If seizures occur, the most likely diagnosis is which of the following?

   a. eclampsia
   b. epilepsy

   c. water intoxication from vasopressin effects of oxytocin
   d. drug reaction

17–26. According to American College of Obstetricians and Gynecologists guidelines, when is failure to progress diagnosed?

   a. The latent phase of labor has been completed.
   b. Montevideo units exceed 200 for 2 hours.
   c. There is no cervical change in 2 hours.
   d. The latent phase of labor exceeds 20 hours.

17–27. Which of the following is NOT a hazard of stripping the membranes?

   a. induction of infection
   b. rupture of membranes
   c. initiating bleeding from a previa
   d. fetal heart rate bradycardia

17–28. In a nulliparous woman, how long is the prolonged deceleration phase?

   a. >1 hr
   b. >2 hr
   c. >3 hr
   d. >20 hr

17–29. Which of the following is NOT associated with precipitate labor and delivery?

   a. amnionic fluid embolism
   b. postpartum hemorrhage
   c. increased perinatal mortality and morbidity
   d. meconium aspiration

17–30. Which of the following is a common postpartum complication of precipitous labor?

   a. hemorrhage
   b. endometritis
   c. mastitis
   d. milk fever

18

Dystocia: Abnormal Presentation, Position, and Development of the Fetus

18–1. What is the approximate incidence of breech presentation at term?

   a. 0.5%
   b. 3.0%
   c. 7.0%
   d. 12.0%

18–2. Which of the following is NOT a risk factor for breech?

   a. multiple fetuses
   b. hydramnios
   c. uterine anomalies
   d. low parity

18–3. Which of the following is NOT associated with persistent breech presentation?

   a. increased perinatal morbidity and mortality
   b. increased macrosomia
   c. increased prolapsed cord
   d. increased placenta previa

18–4. Which of the following describes a frank breech presentation?

   a. flexion of the hips and extension of the knees
   b. flexion of the hips and flexion of the knees
   c. extension of the hips and flexion of the knees
   d. extension of the hips and extension of the knees

18–5. Which of the following best describes the incomplete breech presentation?

   a. lower extremities flexed at the hips and extended at knees
   b. lower extremities flexed at the hips and one or both knees flexed
   c. one or both hips not flexed or both feet or knees below breech
   d. both feet are in the right fundal area

18–6. Which of the following best describes a complete breech presentation?

   a. lower extremities flexed at the hips and extended at knees
   b. lower extremities flexed at the hips and one or both knees flexed
   c. one or both hips not flexed or both feet or knees below breech
   d. a foot in the birth canal

18–7. When examining a woman at term, hearing fetal heart tones loudest above the umbilicus suggests which type of presentation?

   a. cephalic presentation
   b. transverse lie
   c. breech presentation
   d. multiple pregnancy

18–8. At term, what is the most common breech presentation?

   a. frank
   b. complete

c. incomplete
d. footling

18–9. What percentage of breech deliveries will be complicated by nuchal arm?

   a. <1
   b. 3
   c. 6
   d. 10

18–10. Approximately what percentage of breech presentations at term will be associated with an extreme hyperextension of the fetal head?

   a. 0.5
   b. 5.0
   c. 15
   d. 25

18–11. What is the approximate success rate of external cephalic version for breech presentations late in pregnancy?

   a. 25%
   b. 40%
   c. 65%
   d. 90%

18–12. Of successful versions, approximately what percentage will be vertex at delivery?

   a. 40
   b. 67
   c. 80
   d. 97

18–13. Universal application of ECV can reduce the cesarean section by how much?

   a. 10%
   b. 25%
   c. 50%
   d. 80%

18–14. Which of the following may be associated with failure of external cephalic version?

   a. frank breech
   b. anteriorly located fetal spine
   c. ample amnionic fluid
   d. descent of breech into the pelvis

18–15. Which of the following is NOT a complication of external version?

   a. premature labor
   b. fetomaternal hemorrhage
   c. amnionic fluid embolus
   d. placental abruption

18–16. What is the presenting part with a face presentation?

   a. sinciput
   b. malar eminence
   c. mentum
   d. occiput

18–17. Which of the following is NOT associated etiologically with a face presentation?

   a. contracted pelvis
   b. oxytocin induction
   c. macrosomia
   d. pendulous abdomen

18–18. Approximately what percentage of face presentations are associated with inlet contraction?

   a. 5
   b. 20
   c. 40
   d. 65

18–19. In labor, if the presenting part is the sagittal suture midway between the orbital ridge and the anterior fontanelle, what is the presentation?

   a. face
   b. brow
   c. occiput
   d. left occiput anterior

18–20. What bony landmark determines the designation of lie in shoulder presentations?

   a. acromion
   b. brow
   c. breech
   d. occiput

18–21. Which of the following is NOT a common cause of transverse lie?

    a. placenta previa
    b. abnormal uterus
    c. postterm pregnancy
    d. contracted pelvis

18–22. What is the best way to deliver a term transverse lie in labor with ruptured membranes?

    a. low transverse cesarean section
    b. vertical cesarean section
    c. version to vertex and vaginal delivery
    d. version to breech and vaginal delivery

18–23. What is conduplicato corpore?

    a. conjoined twins
    b. position of infant early in pregnancy with delivery of transverse lie
    c. position of the fetus at delivery in which it is doubled upon itself (head and thorax deliver at same time)
    d. a congenital anomaly of the central nervous system

18–24. In the multiparous woman having a fetus with an occiput posterior position, labor is prolonged by approximately how long compared to that of an occiput anterior position?

    a. 30 min
    b. 1 hr
    c. 2 hr
    d. 4 hr

18–25. Of the following methods used for delivery of shoulder dystocia, which is associated with the highest incidence of orthopedic and neurological damage?

    a. suprapubic pressure
    b. McRobert's maneuver
    c. Hibbard's maneuver
    d. Woods screw maneuver

18–26. Which of the following is NOT part of the management of shoulder dystocia?

    a. Woods screw maneuver
    b. fundal pressure
    c. McRobert's maneuver
    d. delivery of posterior shoulder

18–27. What is the incidence of internal hydrocephalus?

    a. 1 in 1000 deliveries
    b. 1 in 2000 deliveries
    c. 1 in 3000 deliveries
    d. 1 in 5000 deliveries

18–28. Which of Leopold's maneuvers is accomplished facing the mother's feet?

    a. 1st
    b. 2nd
    c. 3rd
    d. 4th

19

Dystocia Due to Pelvic Contraction

19–1. What is the shortest AP diameter to be considered pelvic inlet contracture?

    a. <8 cm
    b. <9 cm
    c. <10 cm
    d. <12 cm

19–2. What is the diagonal conjugate generally less than in women with contracted inlet?

    a. 8.0 cm
    b. 9.5 cm
    c. 10.5 cm
    d. 13.0 cm

19–3. What is the average biparietal diameter of term infants?

    a. 8.5 cm
    b. 9.0 cm
    c. 9.5 cm
    d. >10.0 cm

19–4. What is the incidence of shoulder presentation in women who have a contracted inlet compared to normal pelvis?

    a. 2 times more frequently
    b. 3 times more frequently
    c. 4 times more frequently
    d. 6 times more frequently

19–5. Which of the following is NOT a factor associated with fetal head molding?

    a. multiparity
    b. oxytocin labor stimulation
    c. vacuum extractor delivery
    d. prolonged labor

19–6. The midpelvis is likely to be contracted if the sum of the interischial spinous or posterior sagittal diameter is less than what?

    a. 9.5 cm
    b. 11.5 cm
    c. 12.5 cm
    d. 13.5 cm

19–7. In a nullipara at term the diagonal conjugate measures 10.5 cm. Of the following, which is true?

    a. The head is not engaged.
    b. Oxytocin is contraindicated.
    c. Cesarean section is probably necessary.
    d. All of the above are true.

19–8. What is the average interspinous measurement?

    a. 8.0 cm
    b. 9.0 cm
    c. 10.0 cm
    d. 10.5 cm

19–9. What is the average posterior sagittal diameter?

    a. 4 cm
    b. 5 cm
    c. 6 cm
    d. 8 cm

19–10. With what type of presentation is dolichocephaly least common?

    a. breech
    b. twins
    c. vertex
    d. oligohydramnios

19–11. Which of the following factors is amenable to reasonably precise radiographic measurement (x-ray)?

    a. fetal head size
    b. moldability of the fetal head
    c. size of bony pelvis
    d. strength of uterine contractions

19–12. What is the difference between the diagonal conjugate and the obstetrical conjugate?

    a. 1 to 2 cm longer
    b. 3 to 4 cm longer
    c. 1 to 2 cm shorter
    d. both the same size

19–13. Which of the following is NOT an indication for x-ray pelvimetry?

    a. previous cesarean for trial of labor
    b. breech
    c. previous injury to bony pelvis
    d. term failure to progress

19–14. What is the mean gonadal exposure to the fetus with conventional x-ray pelvimetry?

    a. ~0.001 Gy
    b. ~0.01 Gy
    c. ~0.1 Gy
    d. ~1.0 Gy

19–15. What is the average absorbed radiation dose with computed tomograms?

    a. ~0.0002
    b. ~0.002
    c. ~0.02
    d. ~0.2

Operative Obstetrics

20

Operative Vaginal Delivery

20–1. Which of the following is NOT a basic component of a forceps branch?

 a. blade
 b. shank
 c. lock
 d. stem

20–2. Which of the following forceps has parallel shanks?

 a. Tucker–McLane
 b. Simpson
 c. Kielland
 d. Barton

20–3. When forceps are applied to the fetal head in which the scalp is visible at the introitus without separation of the labia, what type of delivery occurs?

 a. outlet forceps
 b. low forceps
 c. midforceps
 d. either outlet or low

20–4. What is the classification for any forceps rotation, including LOA and ROA, at +2 cm or greater?

 a. outlet forceps
 b. low forceps
 c. midforceps
 d. high forceps

20–5. When the fetal head is engaged and at a +1-cm station, how would a forceps delivery be classified?

 a. outlet forceps
 b. low forceps
 c. midforceps
 d. high forceps

20–6. Utilizing the new definitions, forceps applied to the fetal head (LOA) that has reached the pelvic floor when the fetal head is at the perineum should be classified as what type of delivery?

 a. outlet forceps
 b. low forceps
 c. midforceps
 d. high forceps

20–7. Which of the following is NOT associated with regional analgesia?

    a. increased frequency of instrumental delivery

    b. increased frequency of midforceps

    c. increased frequency of occiput posterior positions

    d. decreased frequency of rotational forceps deliveries

20–8. Which of the following forceps is best suited for a low-forceps delivery of a fetus with a molded head?

    a. Simpson

    b. Tucker–McLane

    c. Kielland

    d. Chamberlain

20–9. Which of the following forceps is best suited for a low-forceps delivery of a fetus with a rounded head?

    a. Simpson

    b. Tucker–McLane

    c. Kielland

    d. Chamberlain

20–10. Which of the following maternal conditions is NOT an indication for termination of labor by forceps?

    a. heart disease

    b. acute pulmonary edema

    c. intrapartum infection

    d. second stage of labor of $1\frac{1}{2}$ hr in nullipara

20–11. Which of the following is NOT a fetal indication for termination of labor by forceps?

    a. prolapse of umbilical cord

    b. meconium-stained amnionic fluid

    c. premature separation of placenta

    d. worrisome fetal heart rate pattern

20–12. When exceeded, which of the following is considered a prolonged second stage of labor for the nulliparous patient?

    a. 1 hour without regional anesthesia

    b. 1 hour with regional anesthesia

    c. 2 hours without regional anesthesia

    d. 2 hours with regional anesthesia

20–13. When exceeded, which of the following is the most correct definition of a prolonged second stage in the parous patient?

    a. 1 hour without regional anesthesia

    b. 1 hour with regional anesthesia

    c. 2 hours without regional anesthesia

    d. 2 hours with regional anesthesia

20–14. Forceps should generally NOT be used electively until which of the following criteria is met?

    a. The head is at 0 to +1 station.

    b. The head is at +2 to +3 station.

    c. The head is on the perineal floor.

    d. The head is in an OA position and at least at 0 station.

20–15. With regard to the use of prophylactic forceps, which of the following statements is correct?

    a. They will prevent episiotomy extension.

    b. They will reduce the incidence of fetal brain damage from prolonged perineal pressure.

    c. They are associated with improved neonatal outcome in low birthweight infants.

    d. There is no evidence that they are beneficial in otherwise normal labor and delivery.

20–16. Which of the following is NOT a prerequisite for forceps application?

    a. The head must be engaged.

    b. The fetus must present either by the vertex or by the face with the chin posterior.

    c. The cervix must be completely dilated.

    d. The membranes must be ruptured.

20–17. Which of the following is true concerning the Mueller-Hillis maneuver?

    a. It is an accurate way to determine station.

    b. It does not predict success of forceps delivery.

    c. It is an accurate means to predict dystocia.

    d. It is used to determine engagement.

20–18. Which of the following analgesia/anesthesia techniques is NOT ideal for low-forceps or midpelvic procedures?

    a. pudendal block
    b. spinal block
    c. epidural block
    d. ketamine

20–19. At what point during forceps delivery is the fetal head most likely to be exposed to injurious pressure?

    a. The long axis of the blades correspond to the occipitomental diameter of the fetal head.
    b. The concave margins of the blades are directed toward the sagittal sutures.
    c. The concave margins of the blades are directed toward the face.
    d. The pelvic application is employed.

20–20. Regarding traction with forceps, which of the following statements is incorrect?

    a. Gentle traction should be intermittent.
    b. The fetal head should be allowed to recede in intervals.
    c. Delivery should be deliberate and slow.
    d. It is preferable to apply traction between contractions to avoid excessive pressure.

20–21. Which of the following pelvic architecture is most likely to be associated with occiput transverse positions?

    a. gynecoid
    b. platypelloid
    c. anthropoid
    d. gynecoid–anthropoid combination

20–22. When rotating the fetal head from posterior to anterior positions, it is NOT necessary to flex the head when using which of the forceps below?

    a. Simpson
    b. Tucker-McLane
    c. Simpson-Luikart
    d. Kielland

20–23. Which of the pelvic types is generally associated with the persistent occiput posterior position?

    a. anthropoid
    b. android

    c. platypelloid
    d. gynecoid

20–24. Which of the following is NOT a maternal complication associated with Kielland forceps delivery?

    a. postpartum hemorrhage
    b. protoepisiotomy lacerations
    c. chorioamnionitis
    d. manual removal of the placenta

20–25. Which of the following neonatal morbidities are NOT related to Kielland forceps deliveries?

    a. jaundice
    b. urinary retention
    c. nerve palsies
    d. scalp abscess

20–26. Which of the following is NOT a theoretical advantage of the vacuum extractor over forceps?

    a. not as much vaginal space required
    b. ability to rotate the fetal head without impinging on maternal soft tissues
    c. less intracranial pressure during traction
    d. can be applied at higher stations than forceps

20–27. What is a chignon?

    a. an artificial caput
    b. a scalp hematoma
    c. an abrasion caused by the metal vacuum cup
    d. an abrasion caused by a soft, silastic cup

20–28. Which of the following is NOT a relative contraindication for delivery using vacuum extraction?

    a. face presentation
    b. fetal macrosomia
    c. fetal coagulopathies
    d. postterm pregnancy

20–29. Which of the following is NOT a direct complication of delivery using the vacuum extraction?

    a. cephalohematoma
    b. intracranial hemorrhage
    c. retinal hemorrhage
    d. newborn acidemia

21

Techniques for Breech Delivery

21–1. Which of the following characterizes partial breech extraction?

    a. Infant is expelled entirely to shoulder.
    b. Infant spontaneously delivers to umbilicus.
    c. Infant's buttocks deliver spontaneously.
    d. Infant is extracted by the attendant.

21–2. Which of the following is the best indicator of pelvic adequacy?

    a. normal labor progress
    b. prior 10-lb vaginal delivery
    c. adequate x-ray pelvimetry
    d. position of the breech

21–3. Which procedure involves intrauterine manipulation of a frank breech to a footling breech?

    a. Prague
    b. Pinard
    c. Bracht
    d. breech decomposition

21–4. How should traction in a breech extraction be employed?

    a. parallel to the floor
    b. 30-degree angle toward the ceiling
    c. gentle downward traction
    d. marked downward pull until the axillae are visible

21–5. In which maneuver are the index and middle finger applied over the maxilla in order to free the head?

    a. Pinard
    b. Bracht
    c. Mauriceau–Smellie–Veit
    d. Zavanelli

21–6. With breech delivery, which maneuver is suggested when there is persistence of the fetal spine directed toward the maternal sacrum?

    a. Prague
    b. Bracht
    c. Pinard
    d. Mauriceau–Smellie–Veit

21–7. What is the best position for the operator in applying Piper forceps?

    a. standing
    b. sitting
    c. kneeling on one knee
    d. squatting

21–8. "Abdominal rescue" of a partially delivered breech is similar to which maneuver?

    a. Prague
    b. Zavanelli
    c. Pinard
    d. Bracht

21–9. During early labor in a breech presentation, the fetal heart rate should be evaluated how often?

    a. every 5 min
    b. every 15 min
    c. every 30 min
    d. continuously

21–10. In which of the maneuvers is the fetal body held against the maternal symphysis?

    a. Mauriceau–Smellie–Veit
    b. Bracht
    c. Pinard
    d. Prague

21–11. Which maneuver is employed during a frank breech presentation to deliver the foot into the vagina?

    a. Mauriceau–Smellie–Veit
    b. Bracht
    c. Pinard
    d. Prague

21–12. During a breech delivery, rotation occurs to where the back of the infant is directed toward the maternal vertebral column. If traction occurs, what happens to the fetal head?

    a. It flexes.
    b. It assumes a military position.
    c. It wedges beneath the symphysis.
    d. It extends.

21–13. A 21-year-old, nulliparous D-negative patient at 36 weeks undergoes an external version for breech presentation. Which of the following should be given?

    a. anti-D immunoglobulin
    b. magnesium sulfate
    c. oxytocin
    d. nifedipine

21–14. External version is accomplished at 38 weeks. Which of the following is not a risk?

    a. placental abruption
    b. uterine rupture
    c. induction of labor
    d. fetomaternal hemorrhage

21–15. What is the cost effectiveness of external cephalic version?

    a. marked decrease based on decreased cesarean section
    b. marked increase due to cost of version
    c. marked decrease in multiparas only
    d. not established

21–16. Which of the following is NOT associated with a successful external cephalic version?

    a. frank breech
    b. large amniotic fluid volume
    c. unengaged fetus
    d. parity

22

Cesarean Delivery and Cesarean Hysterectomy

22–1. Which section of the country has the highest cesarean birth rate?

    a. North
    b. South
    c. East
    d. West

22–2. What is the most common indication for a cesarean section in the United States?

    a. fetal distress
    b. breech presentation
    c. dystocia or failure to progress
    d. prior cesarean section

22–3. In the United States, what is the most common indication for a primary cesarean section?

   a. fetal distress
   b. breech presentation
   c. dystocia or failure to progress
   d. macrosomia

22–4. In the United States what percentage of fetuses presenting as breech are delivered by cesarean section?

   a. 25
   b. 38
   c. 75
   d. 83

22–5. What is the incidence of uterine rupture in women with prior classical cesareans given a trial of labor?

   a. 1%
   b. 6%
   c. 12%
   d. 20%

22–6. An uneventful trial of labor is in progress in a woman with a previous cesarean section. Sudden persistent bradycardia most likely represents which of the following?

   a. cord occlusion
   b. rupture of the uterus
   c. placental abruption
   d. hyperstimulation

22–7. Which of the following is an absolute contraindication to trial of labor with a previous cesarean section?

   a. two prior transverse cesarean births
   b. oxytocin
   c. prior classical cesarean section
   d. prior dystocia

22–8. What is the expected success rate for vaginal delivery in women with prior cesarean undergoing trial of labor?

   a. 30%
   b. 50%
   c. 70%
   d. 90%

22–9. Which of the following is true concerning planned vaginal breech delivery compared to planned cesarean births?

   a. a 4-fold increase in perinatal mortality
   b. a 2-fold increase in perinatal mortality
   c. no change in perinatal mortality
   d. a slight but insignificant increase in perinatal mortality

22–10. What is the least common type of cesarean section?

   a. Frank–Latzko
   b. Kerr–Munro
   c. Krönig
   d. classical

22–11. Which of the following is NOT an advantage of low transverse cesarean deliveries?

   a. easier to repair
   b. less blood loss
   c. less problems with adhesions from bowel
   d. ability to safely extend incision laterally

22–12. Which of the following is an advantage of the transverse skin incision?

   a. exposure of uterus and appendages
   b. easy to extend incision rapidly
   c. stronger than a vertical incision
   d. less hematoma formation subfascially

22–13. Which of the following is true when the uterine incision is repaired with vicryl?

   a. increased adhesion to bowel
   b. increased scar separation
   c. decreased blood loss
   d. decreased infection

22–14. Which of the following is NOT an indication for a classical cesarean incision?

   a. cannot visualize the lower segment
   b. transverse lie
   c. premature breech
   d. term breech (frank)

22–15. What is the average blood loss with a cesarean hysterectomy?

   a. 500 mL
   b. 1000 mL

c. 1500 mL
d. 3000 mL

22–16. What is the approximate rate for rupture of the uterus from all causes?

a. <0.1%
b. <1.0%
c. 3 to 5%
d. 10 to 12%

22–17. Which of the following is NOT associated with uterine rupture?

a. separation of incision throughout its length
b. fetus extruded into peritoneal cavity
c. bleeding
d. ruptured membranes

22–18. What is the MOST common finding with uterine rupture?

a. change in intrauterine pressure readings
b. sudden tearing abdominal pain
c. fetal distress
d. signs of hemorrhage

22–19. The cesarean section rate in the United States has stabilized at approximately what percentage?

a. 10
b. 25
c. 33
d. 50

22–20. Which of the following is associated with reducing the cesarean section rate?

a. vaginal delivery of breech presentation
b. changing the legal nonsystem
c. vaginal birth after cesarean section
d. discontinuing electronic fetal monitoring

22–21. Which of the following is NOT associated with prophylactic antibiotic failure?

a. number of vaginal exams
b. nulliparity
c. postterm gestation
d. use of cefazolin

Abnormalities of the Puerperium

$$\boxed{23}$$

The Puerperium

23–1. What is the anterior uterine wall thickness immediately after expulsion of the placenta?

  a. <1 cm
  b. 2 to 3 cm
  c. 4 to 5 cm
  d. 8 cm

23–2. At what time postpartum does the uterus return to its nonpregnant size?

  a. 2 weeks
  b. 4 weeks
  c. 6 weeks
  d. 12 weeks

23–3. By what time postpartum is the endometrium restored?

  a. 1 week
  b. 2 weeks
  c. 3 weeks
  d. 4 weeks

23–4. How long does it take for complete extrusion of the placental bed?

  a. 2 weeks
  b. 4 weeks
  c. 6 weeks
  d. 12 weeks

23–5. Placental site exfoliation is brought about by what process?

  a. hypertrophic repair
  b. decrease in myometrial cell size
  c. proliferation of new endometrial glands
  d. necrotic sloughing

23–6. Which of the following are characteristics of the puerperal bladder?

  a. underdistension; complete emptying
  b. underdistension; incomplete emptying
  c. overdistension; complete emptying
  d. overdistension; incomplete emptying

23–7. Which is NOT associated with postpartum stress urinary incontinence?

  a. prolonged second stage
  b. size of infant's head
  c. episiotomy
  d. cesarean section

23–8. At what time in the puerperium do the renal pelvises and ureters return to prepregnant size?

    a. 1 day
    b. 5 days
    c. 10 days
    d. 2 to 8 weeks

23–9. Which breast cell type synthesizes milk?

    a. secretory epithelium
    b. mucous epithelium
    c. myoepithelium
    d. glandular cell

23–10. During thelarche, which hormone stimulates development of the alveoli?

    a. estrogen
    b. cortisol
    c. progesterone
    d. growth hormone

23–11. Compared to breast milk, colostrum contains more of which of the following?

    a. fat
    b. minerals
    c. sugar
    d. immunoglobulin M

23–12. Which of the following factors has NOT been identified in breast milk?

    a. interleukin-6
    b. prolactin
    c. epidermal growth factor
    d. somatostatin

23–13. Which vitamin is NOT found in breast milk?

    a. vitamin B
    b. vitamin C
    c. vitamin D
    d. vitamin K

23–14. Which of the following is concentrated in breast milk?

    a. iron
    b. iodine
    c. chloride
    d. riboflavin

23–15. Which hormone is responsible for causing contractions in myoepithelial cells?

    a. oxytocin
    b. prolactin
    c. progesterone
    d. placental lactogen

23–16. Which of the following is a direct benefit of breastfeeding to the newborn?

    a. increase in protein
    b. increase in vitamin D
    c. decrease in enteric infection
    d. decrease in fat content

23–17. How do oral contraceptives inhibit the mechanism of lactation?

    a. block milk secretion
    b. decrease the volume of milk produced
    c. inhibit milk release
    d. block secretion of oxytocin

23–18. Which of the following maternal infections is NOT a contraindication to breastfeeding?

    a. cytomegalovirus
    b. chronic hepatitis B
    c. human immunodeficiency virus infection
    d. herpes simplex infection of the cervix

23–19. Which of the following drugs is concentrated in human milk?

    a. bromocriptine
    b. cocaine
    c. doxorubicin
    d. lithium

23–20. What is the order of the stages of lochia (beginning with early postpartum)?

    a. lochia rubra, lochia alba, lochia serosa
    b. lochia rubra, lochia serosa, lochia alba
    c. lochia serosa, lochia alba, lochia rubra
    d. lochia alba, lochia serosa, lochia rubra

23–21. Most women return to their prepregnancy weight by what time postpartum?

    a. 2 months
    b. 3 months
    c. 4 months
    d. 6 months

23–22. In general, where should the uterus be palpable postpartum?

    a. below umbilicus
    b. at umbilicus
    c. above umbilicus
    d. above symphysis

23–23. Which of the following is recommended to minimize episiotomy discomfort immediately postpartum?

    a. codeine 30 mg every 8 hr
    b. morphine 10 mg every 2 hr
    c. aspirin 600 mg every 8 hr
    d. ice packs to perineum

23–24. Which of the following is prominent in the genesis of "postpartum blues"?

    a. the excitement of pregnancy
    b. the discomforts of the early puerperium
    c. the rest obtained in the hospital
    d. comfort over taking care of the child

23–25. Which of the following immunizations should NOT be given postpartum?

    a. diphtheria–tetanus
    b. anti-D immune globulin

    c. hepatitis B
    d. no restrictions for any that are indicated

23–26. By what time postpartum are infection and hemorrhage less likely and therefore coitus may resume?

    a. 3 to 4 days
    b. 7 to 10 days
    c. 14 to 21 days
    d. 28 to 30 days

23–27. At what point postpartum does menstruation normally return in a nonbreastfeeding woman?

    a. 1 to 2 weeks
    b. 3 to 4 weeks
    c. 6 to 8 weeks
    d. 12 weeks or later

23–28. Which hormone is lower in lactating women?

    a. luteinizing hormone
    b. growth hormone
    c. prolactin
    d. cortisol

24

Infection and Other Disorders of the Puerperium

24–1. What is the maternal mortality ratio owing to infection?

    a. 0.06 per 100,000 live births
    b. 0.6 per 100,000 live births
    c. 6 per 100,000 live births
    d. 6 per 100,000 pregnancies

24–2. What is the definition of puerperal morbidity?

    a. temperature of 38.0°C (104°F) or greater after day 1
    b. temperature of 38.0°C or greater on day 1
    c. temperature of 37.5°C or greater
    d. temperature of 39°C on day 1

24–3. Which of the following organisms is associated with high fevers in the first 24 hours after childbirth?

    a. group A streptococcus
    b. *Bacteroides bivius*
    c. *Peptostreptococcus*
    d. *Bacteroides fragilis*

24–4. How can the frequency of atelectasis be decreased?

    a. by coughing and deep breathing
    b. by deep breathing and taking aspirin
    c. by not using morphine for pain control postoperatively
    d. by giving theophylline prophylactically

24–5. Fever owing to breast engorgement is self-limited and generally, at the most, lasts how long?

    a. one temperature elevation
    b. 24 hr
    c. 48 hr
    d. 72 hr

24–6. What is the single most significant risk factor for postpartum metritis?

    a. number of pelvic exams
    b. duration of labor
    c. duration of amniorrhexis
    d. route of delivery

24–7. Which of the following is NOT considered a high-risk factor for metritis?

    a. prolonged labor and ruptured membranes
    b. internal monitoring
    c. cephalopelvic disproportion
    d. preterm labor

24–8. Which of the following in serum may have significant antibacterial action?

    a. increased serum iron
    b. increased serum transferrin
    c. increased serum folate
    d. increased serum B_{12}

24–9. Which of the following lower genital tract organisms is not associated with increased postpartum infection?

    a. *Trichomonas vaginalis*
    b. group B streptococcus
    c. *Gardnerella vaginalis*
    d. *Mycoplasma hominis*

24–10. Which of the following organisms has been associated with toxic shock-like syndrome?

    a. *Staphylococcus epidermidis*
    b. *E. coli*
    c. group A β-hemolytic streptococcus
    d. *Klebsiella pneumoniae*

24–11. Which of the following bacteria is anaerobic?

    a. *Enterococcus* sp.
    b. group A streptococcus
    c. *Staphylococcus aureus*
    d. *Clostridium* sp.

24–12. Which of the following is characteristic of uterine infections?

    a. anaerobic
    b. aerobic
    c. monoetiology
    d. polymicrobial

24–13. Which of the following organisms is implicated as a cause of late postpartum infection?

    a. *N. gonorrhoeae*
    b. *C. trachomatis*
    c. *T. vaginalis*
    d. *B. bivius*

24–14. Blood cultures are positive in what percentage of women with postpartum metritis?

    a. <0.1
    b. 1 to 2
    c. 8 to 10
    d. >10

24–15. Which of the following does not favor anaerobic bacterial growth?

    a. surgical trauma
    b. lymphatic drainage
    c. devitalized tissue
    d. collection of blood and serum

24–16. Which of the following puerperal infections is associated with scanty, odorless lochia?

a. *Chlamydia trachomatis*
b. *N. gonorrhoeae*
c. *Enterococcus* sp.
d. group A β-hemolytic streptococci

24–17. What percentage of cases of puerperal metritis will respond to antimicrobials within 72 hours?

a. 25
b. 50
c. 75
d. 90

24–18. How long should women with puerperal metritis be treated with antimicrobials?

a. until afebrile for 24 hours
b. for a 5-day course
c. for a 10-day course
d. for a 14-day course

24–19. Which of the following is a β-lactamase inhibitor?

a. sodium salt
b. acetic acid
c. clavulanic acid
d. sodium citrate

24–20. Which of the following antibiotic regimens is considered the "gold standard" therapy for puerperal metritis?

a. ampicillin plus gentamicin
b. gentamicin plus clindamycin
c. ampicillin plus clindamycin
d. ampicillin plus gentamicin plus clindamycin

24–21. Which of the following is recommended therapy for pseudomembranous colitis?

a. vibramycin
b. methicillin
c. clindamycin
d. metronidazole

24–22. In the presence of an abscess, which of the following agents is recommended?

a. chloramphenicol
b. metronidazole
c. aztreonam
d. ticarcillin

24–23. Which of the following inhibits the renal metabolism of imipenem?

a. clavulanic acid
b. sulbactam
c. aztreonam
d. cilastatin

24–24. Which of the following is a carbapenem?

a. carbenicillin
b. imipenem
c. ticarcillin
d. primaxin

24–25. Following cesarean section, prophylactic antibiotics decrease the incidence of abdominal incisional infection from 7 percent to what?

a. 5%
b. 2%
c. 1%
d. <0.1%

24–26. Which of the following is NOT a risk factor for necrotizing fasciitis?

a. obesity
b. hypertension
c. diabetes
d. anemia

24–27. When compared with surgical peritonitis, puerperal peritonitis has less of which of the following?

a. bowel distention
b. abdominal rigidity
c. pain
d. all of the above

24–28. What is a parametrial phlegmon?

a. an ovarian abscess
b. a pelvic abscess in the Pouch of Douglas
c. a tubal abscess
d. an induration from cellulitis within the leaves of the broad ligament

24–29. Which of the following characterizes the examination in a woman with a phlegmon?

a. fixed uterus pushed contralateral to phlegmon
b. fixed uterus pushed ipsilateral to phlegmon
c. marked abdominal distention
d. absent bowel sounds

24–30. What is the recommended treatment of a parametrial phlegmon?

    a. antibiotics alone
    b. heparin plus antibiotics
    c. hysterectomy
    d. percutaneous drainage

24–31. What percentage of women with refractory pelvic infections will have abnormal radiographic findings (i.e., computed tomography)?

    a. 5 to 10
    b. 20 to 25
    c. 50 to 60
    d. >75

24–32. What is the management of choice for a rectovaginal septal abscess?

    a. antibiotics only
    b. computed tomographic needle drainage
    c. posterior colpotomy
    d. total abdominal hysterectomy

24–33. What is the cause of septic vein thrombophlebitis?

    a. aerobic infection
    b. anaerobic infection
    c. *Streptococcus clotiza*
    d. *Bacteroides thrombotica*

24–34. To where will severe septic phlebitis of the left ovarian vein extend?

    a. vena cava
    b. left renal vein
    c. common iliac veins
    d. internal iliac

24–35. What is the clinical pathognomonic feature of a woman with septic thrombophlebitis?

    a. fever
    b. lower abdominal pain
    c. leg pain
    d. distended abdomen

24–36. What is the cardinal symptom of ovarian vein thrombophlebitis?

    a. fever
    b. lower abdominal pain
    c. leg pain
    d. no symptoms

24–37. Which of the following is the best test for pelvic phlebitis?

    a. the heparin challenge test
    b. ultrasound
    c. magnetic resonance imaging
    d. abdominal x-ray

24–38. What is the approximate incidence of episiotomy breakdown?

    a. 0.1%
    b. 0.5%
    c. 1.0%
    d. 5.0%

24–39. What is the most common etiology of episiotomy breakdown?

    a. poor nutrition
    b. devascularization
    c. failure to reapproximate tissues adequately
    d. infection

24–40. Of the following which is NOT a clinical finding in episiotomy infection?

    a. red, brawny wound edges
    b. lymphangitis
    c. edema
    d. serosanguineous exudates

24–41. Early repair of episiotomy breakdown is successful in what percentage of patients?

    a. <15
    b. 20 to 30
    c. 50 to 60
    d. >90

24–42. Which of the following organisms predominate in necrotizing fasciitis?

    a. aerobic organisms
    b. anaerobic organisms
    c. fungi
    d. chlamydia

24–43. Which of the following is NOT recommended for the immediate treatment of necrotizing fasciitis?

    a. broad-spectrum antibiotics
    b. aggressive surgical debridement
    c. split-thickness skin grafts
    d. fascial debridement

24–44. What is the case–fatality rate for toxic shock syndrome?

   a. 1%
   b. 10%
   c. 20%
   d. 50%

24–45. Which of the following organisms is responsible for toxic shock syndrome?

   a. *Staphylococcus aureus*
   b. *Staphylococcus epidermidis*
   c. *Staphylococcus pyrogenes*
   d. *Staphylococcus toxi*

24–46. Which of the following toxins is responsible for the profound endothelial injury in toxic shock syndrome?

   a. endotoxin
   b. hypogenic exotoxin
   c. pyodermic toxin
   d. toxic shock syndrome toxin-1

24–47. Approximately what percentage of late postpartum uterine infections are caused by *Chlamydia trachomatis?*

   a. 2
   b. 15
   c. 33
   d. 50

24–48. Approximately what percentage of women will develop significant uterine bleeding after the first 24 hours postpartum?

   a. <1
   b. 5 to 6
   c. 10
   d. 17

24–49. Approximately what percentage of postpartum women will manifest transient fever from breast engorgement?

   a. <1
   b. 15
   c. 25
   d. 35

24–50. For what reason was postpartum lactation suppression deleted from indications for bromocriptine?

   a. hypertension
   b. seizures
   c. myocardial infarction
   d. all of the above

24–51. According to the Food and Drug Administration, which of the following drugs should be utilized for routine suppression of breast engorgement?

   a. estrogen
   b. estrogen plus testosterone
   c. bromocriptine
   d. none

24–52. Approximately what percentage of women with mastitis will develop a breast abscess?

   a. <1
   b. 5
   c. 10
   d. 20

24–53. What is the most common etiologic agent for mastitis?

   a. *Staphylococcus aureus*
   b. *Staphylococcus epidermitis*
   c. enterococci
   d. group A streptococci

24–54. What is the treatment of choice for a postpartum breast abscess?

   a. vancomycin
   b. doxycycline
   c. surgical drainage
   d. erythromycin

24–55. What is the recurrence risk of postpartum psychosis in subsequent pregnancies?

   a. 5%
   b. 25%
   c. 50%
   d. 80%

Reproductive Success and Failure

$\boxed{25}$

Pregnancy at the Extremes of Reproductive Life

25–1. What percentage of U.S. births occur in teenagers or women over 35 years of age?

 a. 10
 b. 25
 c. 33
 d. 50

25–2. In regard to older teenagers (16 to 18 years of age), which of the following is NOT considered to be an obstetrical risk?

 a. physiological immaturity
 b. poverty
 c. inadequate nutrition
 d. poor health before pregnancy

25–3. Increasing birth rates for women under 20 years of age correlate best with which of the following?

 a. increasing sexually transmitted diseases
 b. increasing sexual activity
 c. parental permissiveness
 d. declining influence of the church

25–4. What is the mean age of menarche in the United States?

 a. 9.6 years
 b. 10.4 years
 c. 12.8 years
 d. 13.9 years

25–5. What is the major etiology of teenage maternal mortality?

 a. hemorrhage
 b. infection
 c. hypertension
 d. all of the above

25–6. Preterm birth and pregnancy-induced hypertension in teenagers are significantly increased owing to which of the following?

 a. certain racial characteristics
 b. the mother's social status
 c. middle school-age mothers (age <15)
 d. high school-age mothers (ages 15 to 18)

25–7. Which of the following is frequently associated with teenage pregnancy?

    a. maternal mortality
    b. perinatal mortality
    c. feelings of failure
    d. suicide

25–8. What is the incidence of unintended pregnancy in the United States?

    a. 10%
    b. 25%
    c. 33%
    d. 50%

25–9. With the advancing age of first pregnancy, which of the following is most likely true?

    a. Chronic hypertension is increased.
    b. Preeclampsia is increased.
    c. Preeclampsia is decreased.
    d. Chronic hypertension is decreased.

25–10. Compared with younger women, what is the maternal mortality ratio in women over 35 years of age?

    a. the same
    b. increased 4-fold
    c. increased 8-fold
    d. increased 10-fold

25–11. What happens to abortion rates with advanced maternal age?

    a. remain the same
    b. increase slightly
    c. increase 4-fold
    d. increase 8-fold

25–12. What happens to the preterm birth rate in older women?

    a. decreases
    b. stays the same
    c. increases 2-fold
    d. increases 4-fold

25–13. What is the incidence of aneuploidy in women at age 40 years?

    a. 1 in 200
    b. 1 in 100
    c. 1 in 50
    d. 1 in 25

26

Abortion

26–1. For how long are ejaculated spermatozoa capable of fertilization?

    a. 6 hr
    b. 12 hr
    c. 24 hr
    d. 48 hr

26–2. What is the optimum time for fertilization of the ovum?

    a. 1 to 2 hours after ovulation
    b. 2 to 4 hours after ovulation
    c. 4 to 6 hours after ovulation
    d. 6 to 8 hours after ovulation

26–3. In healthy fertile women, what is the percentage of abortion in clinically recognized pregnancies in the first trimester?

   a. 5
   b. 10
   c. 15
   d. 20

26–4. How often does anovulation occur in young, fertile women on the average?

   a. once every 3 months
   b. once every 7 months
   c. once every 13 months
   d. once every 21 months

26–5. After an abortion, when does ovulation usually occur?

   a. at 2 to 3 weeks
   b. at 4 to 5 weeks
   c. at 5 to 6 weeks
   d. at 6 to 7 weeks

26–6. Which of the following is NOT associated with an increased abortion rate?

   a. advanced maternal age
   b. advanced paternal age
   c. pregnancy within 3 months of a live birth
   d. class A_1 diabetes mellitus

26–7. In first trimester abortions, what is the most common chromosomal anomaly?

   a. triploidy
   b. autosomal trisomy
   c. tetraploidy
   d. structural anomaly

26–8. Which of the following is NOT associated with euploid abortions?

   a. 16th week gestation
   b. maternal age
   c. maternal disease
   d. advanced paternal age

26–9. Of the following, which is most likely to cause abortion?

   a. *Toxoplasma gondii*
   b. *Listeria monocytogenes*
   c. *Chlamydia trachomatis*
   d. *Brucella abortus*

26–10. What is the incidence of abortion in diabetics compared to the general population?

   a. increased
   b. decreased
   c. the same
   d. related to glucose control

26–11. Luteal phase defect is best diagnosed by which of the following?

   a. progesterone level below 9 ng/mL on day 14
   b. luteinizing hormone level below 9 ng/mL on day 14
   c. estradiol excretion below 15 mg/24 hr
   d. estriol excretion below 15 mg/24 hr

26–12. Of the following, which is NOT associated with an increased abortion rate?

   a. tobacco
   b. oral contraceptives
   c. radiation over 5 rads
   d. coffee in excess of 4 cups per day

26–13. Of the following, which is NOT associated with an increased risk of abortion?

   a. diagnostic x-ray
   b. lead
   c. benzene
   d. ethylene oxide

26–14. Which of the following is NOT true regarding the lupus anticoagulant?

   a. It causes vascular damage.
   b. It causes a prolonged activated partial thromboplastin time.
   c. It is both IgG and IgM.
   d. It is associated with an increased risk of postpartum hemorrhage.

26–15. Which of the following tests is best to confirm the lupus anticoagulant?

   a. factor VIII assay
   b. factor VIIa assay
   c. prolonged dilute Russel viper venom time
   d. platelet aggregation studies

26–16. How is an incompetent cervix most frequently diagnosed?

   a. sonography
   b. passage of a #8 Hegar dilator through the internal os
   c. history
   d. hysterography

26–17. What is the approximate success rate following cerclage?

   a. 15%
   b. 30%
   c. 60%
   d. 90%

26–18. At 8 weeks' gestation if vaginal bleeding occurs, what is the risk of spontaneous abortion?

   a. 10%
   b. 30%
   c. 50%
   d. 70%

26–19. Which of the following is associated with bleeding at 8 weeks' gestation?

   a. preterm labor
   b. low birthweight
   c. neonatal mortality
   d. malformations

26–20. At 8 weeks' gestation a woman has bleeding, and an intrauterine device suture is visible at the external os. Because the woman desires to keep the pregnancy, what is the best plan of management?

   a. bed rest
   b. antibiotics
   c. progesterone
   d. removal of the intrauterine device

26–21. At 8 weeks' gestation a woman has vaginal bleeding of supracervical origin. Which of the following is NOT helpful in regard to prognosis?

   a. chorionic gonadotropin
   b. plasma estriol
   c. serum progesterone
   d. ultrasound

26–22. In a woman with three or more recurrent spontaneous abortions, which of the following is NOT true?

   a. The risk of abortion with the next pregnancy is about one-third.
   b. With a successful pregnancy, the risk of preterm delivery is increased.
   c. Parental karyotyping is recommended.
   d. Artificial insemination is almost always successful.

26–23. In the process of very high-dose oxytocin infusion to induce an abortion in the mid-trimester a woman has a seizure. Which laboratory test would be most valuable in diagnosis?

   a. serum magnesium level
   b. serum calcium level
   c. serum sodium level
   d. serum potassium level

26–24. Which of the following is true regarding RU486 (mifepristone)?

   a. causes severe malformations
   b. is most effective prior to 6 weeks' gestation
   c. devoid of side effects
   d. almost 100 percent effective when used as an abortifacient

26–25. What famous case established the legality of elective abortion in the United States?

   a. Jones vs. Smith
   b. Harris vs. Harper
   c. Roe vs. Wade
   d. Anonymous vs. United States

27

Ectopic Pregnancy

27–1. Tubal pregnancies are increased in all but which of the following?

   a. salpingitis
   b. tubal anomalies
   c. previous ectopic pregnancy
   d. abnormal embryos

27–2. Which describes the risk of an ectopic pregnancy after two induced abortions?

   a. decreased
   b. doubled
   c. tripled
   d. unchanged

27–3. Of the following, which may be a functional factor contributing to ectopic pregnancy?

   a. progestin-only oral contraceptive
   b. intrauterine device
   c. postovulatory estrogen (morning-after pill)
   d. all of the above

27–4. Ectopic pregnancy has been reported to be increased with which of the following assisted reproductive techniques?

   a. ovulation induction
   b. gamete intrafallopian transfer (GIFT)
   c. in vitro fertilization (IVF)
   d. all of the above

27–5. Which method of contraceptive failure has the highest ectopic rate?

   a. intrauterine device
   b. oral contraception
   c. tubal sterilization
   d. hysterectomy

27–6. What is the mortality from ectopic pregnancy?

   a. an actual decrease in the number of deaths
   b. a decrease in the percentage of maternal mortality
   c. a case fatality rate increase
   d. all of the above

27–7. What is the most common ectopic tubal implantation site?

   a. fimbria
   b. ampulla
   c. isthmus
   d. cornua

27–8. Which describes the Arias–Stella reaction?

   a. It is specific for ectopic gestation.
   b. It may be confused with a malignancy.
   c. It is specific for intrauterine gestation.
   d. It is the result of unopposed estrogen.

27–9. Which of the following is true about interstitial pregnancy?

   a. represents 3 percent of tubal pregnancies
   b. frequently diagnosed later (8 to 16 weeks)
   c. usually associated with massive hemorrhage with rupture
   d. all of the above

27–10. What is the most common symptom of ectopic pregnancy?

   a. bleeding
   b. pain
   c. dizziness
   d. gastrointestinal symptoms

27–11. Which is the most sensitive pregnancy test?

    a. latex agglutination inhibition slide test
    b. latex agglutination inhibition tube test
    c. enzyme-linked immunosorbent assay (ELISA)
    d. serum chorionic gonadotropin assay (β-hCG)

27–12. A patient with a positive pregnancy test and amenorrhea with a serum progesterone of 5 ng/mL is suggestive of which of the following?

    a. an ectopic pregnancy
    b. an intrauterine pregnancy
    c. a lifeless pregnancy
    d. none of the above

27–13. Using abdominal ultrasound, when can an intrauterine gestational sac be reliably seen?

    a. 7 days postconception
    b. 14 days postconception
    c. 21 days postconception
    d. 28 days postconception

27–14. What is the mean doubling time for β-hCG in early pregnancy?

    a. 24 hr
    b. 48 hr
    c. 72 hr
    d. 96 hr

27–15. Following resection of an ectopic pregnancy, serum chorionic gonadotropin is usually NOT detectable at what point?

    a. 2 days
    b. 4 days
    c. 8 days
    d. 12 days

27–16. In consideration of methotrexate for therapy of an ectopic pregnancy, which of the following would make this choice unwise?

    a. pregnancy of 6 weeks' duration
    b. tubal mass 3.5 cm
    c. fetal heart motion
    d. a primigravida patient

27–17. What is the failure rate of methotrexate therapy for an ectopic pregnancy?

    a. 1%
    b. 3%
    c. 7%
    d. 15%

27–18. What is the status of tubal patency following therapy with methotrexate for an ectopic pregnancy compared with surgery?

    a. decreased
    b. unchanged
    c. increased
    d. unknown

27–19. Which of the following hormones has been injected into the tube for treatment of ectopic pregnancy?

    a. estradiol-17β
    b. progesterone
    c. prostaglandin $F_{2\alpha}$
    d. testosterone

27–20. How is abdominal pregnancy best diagnosed?

    a. x-ray
    b. oxytocin challenge test
    c. physical examination
    d. ultrasound

27–21. Which of the following is a component of Spiegelberg criteria for ovarian pregnancy?

    a. Intact tube is on the affected side.
    b. Fetal sac occupies position of the ovary.
    c. The ovarian ligament must connect the uterus and ovary.
    d. all of the above.

27–22. What is the best method of therapy for a cervical pregnancy?

    a. hysterectomy
    b. cerclage
    c. embolization
    d. chemotherapy with methotrexate

28

Abnormalities of the Reproductive Tract

28–1. Which of the following is commonly associated with Müllerian duct deformities?

    a. cardiac anomalies
    b. renal anomalies
    c. gastrointestinal tract abnormalities
    d. limb anomalies

28–2. Hysteroscopic therapy is best utilized for which uterine anomaly?

    a. bicornuate uterus
    b. septate uterus
    c. uterine didelphys
    d. unicornuate uterus

28–3. Which of the following is associated with the worst pregnancy outcomes?

    a. unicornuate uterus
    b. bicornuate uterus
    c. septate uterus
    d. uterus didelphys

28–4. During gestation, when do the metanephric ducts connect with the cloaca?

    a. 3rd and 5th weeks
    b. 6th and 8th weeks
    c. 10th and 14th weeks
    d. 18th and 20th weeks

28–5. At which gestational week is the uterus formed by the union of two Müllerian ducts?

    a. 3
    b. 6
    c. 10
    d. 15

28–6. What causes a transverse vaginal septum?

    a. defective midline fusion of Müllerian ducts
    b. defective canalization of the vagina
    c. absent midline fusion
    d. incomplete resorption of tissue between the two fused Müllerian ducts

28–7. What is the sensitivity of ultrasound screening for uterine anomalies?

    a. 5%
    b. 20%
    c. 40%
    d. 90%

28–8. What percentage of women with Müllerian defects have associated auditory defects?

    a. <1
    b. 15
    c. 33
    d. 55

28–9. In the presence of a uterine septum, which of the following pregnancy complications is increased?

    a. fetal growth retardation
    b. rudimentary horn pregnancy
    c. ectopic pregnancy
    d. abortion

28–10. What is the most common pregnancy complication in a woman with a unicornuate uterus?

    a. ectopic pregnancy
    b. abortion
    c. preterm delivery
    d. fetal growth retardation

28–11. Prophylactic cervical cerclages are indicated for women with which condition?

   a. unicornuate uterus
   b. septate uterus
   c. transvaginal septum
   d. all of the above

28–12. What is the best method of repair of a bicornuate uterus?

   a. hysteroscopic resection
   b. transvaginal metroplasty
   c. transabdominal metroplasty
   d. laparoscopic metroplasty

28–13. What percentage of women exposed to DES in utero have identifiable structural variations in the cervix and vagina?

   a. <1
   b. 10
   c. 25 to 50
   d. 66 to 75

28–14. During pregnancy Bartholin's abscesses are caused by *Neisseria gonorrhoeae* in what percentage of cases?

   a. 10
   b. 20
   c. 40
   d. 80

28–15. Which therapy for condyloma accuminata during pregnancy is probably contraindicated?

   a. laser
   b. trichloracetic acid
   c. α-interferon
   d. cautery

28–16. Cervical stenosis diagnosed during labor is most commonly the result of which of the following?

   a. congenital abnormalities
   b. female circumcision
   c. conization of the cervix
   d. carcinoma of the cervix

28–17. Symptoms of an incarcerated retroflexed uterus include which of the following?

   a. inability to void
   b. lower abdominal pain

   c. azotemia
   d. all of the above

28–18. In a woman at term and in labor, an elongated vagina passing above the level of the fetal head likely represents which of the following?

   a. Bandl's refraction ring
   b. rupture of the uterus
   c. sacculation
   d. the presence of a leiomyoma

28–19. During pregnancy, a 20-cm myoma is noted. It is followed throughout pregnancy, and the size does not change. This is likely due to which of the following?

   a. red degeneration
   b. decreased estrogen receptors
   c. increased epidermal growth factor
   d. increased progesterone receptors

28–20. What is the best pregnancy management of a 28-year-old nullipara who undergoes a myomectomy in which the endometrial cavity was entered?

   a. labor allowed
   b. onset of labor allowed, then cesarean section
   c. cesarean section near term prior to labor
   d. oxytocin induction at 38 weeks

28–21. What is the most frequent and serious complication of benign ovarian cysts during pregnancy?

   a. malignant transformation
   b. rupture
   c. torsion
   d. dystocia

28–22. What are the two most common neoplasms found in pregnancy?

   a. corpus luteum cyst and benign cystic teratomas
   b. corpus luteum cysts and mucinous cystadenoma
   c. benign cystic teratomas and mucinous cystadenomas
   d. benign cystic teratomas and fibroma

28–23. What is the best management for a patient with a simple cyst measuring 8 cm that is found on pelvic examination and sonography during the 8th week of pregnancy?

    a. immediate laparotomy
    b. laparotomy at 16 to 20 weeks
    c. observation and serial sonography
    d. laparoscopic evaluation with drainage of cyst

28–24. A fetal sonographic study and amniotic fluid alphafetoprotein are normal, but an elevated serum alphafetoprotein is noted at 16 weeks. What might this represent?

    a. mucinous cystadenoma
    b. benign cystic teratoma

    c. dysgerminoma
    d. endodermal sinus tumor

28–25. What is the best course of action for a complex 12-cm adnexal mass noted at 18 weeks' gestation?

    a. observation
    b. laparotomy after delivery
    c. immediate laparotomy
    d. sonographically directed aspiration

Placental Disorders

29

Diseases and Abnormalities of the Fetal Membranes

29–1. At what gestational age is meconium passage uncommon?

   a. <36 weeks
   b. <38 weeks
   c. <40 weeks
   d. <42 weeks

29–2. What is the approximate incidence of meconium-stained amnionic fluid near term?

   a. 0.1%
   b. 1.0%
   c. 10%
   d. 50%

29–3. Which of the following is associated with meconium-stained amniotic fluid?

   a. increased perinatal mortality
   b. vaginal delivery
   c. alkalemia
   d. chorioamnionitis

29–4. What is the histological finding in chorioamnionitis?

   a. plasma cells and mononuclear cells
   b. plasma cells and polymorphonuclear leukocytes
   c. mononuclear cells and polymorphonuclear leukocytes
   d. mononuclear cells and lymphocytes

29–5. What is the composition of amnionic caruncles?

   a. vernix and ectodermal debris
   b. mononuclear cells and macrophages
   c. lymphocytes and polymorphonucleocytes
   d. eosinophils and vernix

29–6. What congenital anomaly is associated with amnion nodosum?

   a. ventral septal defect
   b. spina bifida
   c. omphalocele
   d. hypoplastic kidneys

29–7. At what point in normal gestation should the amnionic fluid volume be approximately 1000 mL?

a. 16 weeks
b. 28 weeks
c. 36 weeks
d. 40 weeks

29–8. Polyhydramnios is an amnionic fluid volume greater than which of the following?

a. 1200 mL
b. 1600 mL
c. 2000 mL
d. 2400 mL

29–9. Which of the following amniotic fluid indices is considered hydramnios?

a. 20
b. 24
c. 28
d. 32

29–10. Which of the following anomalies are not associated with polyhydramnios?

a. central nervous system abnormalities
b. duodenal atresia
c. esophageal atresia
d. renal agenesis

29–11. What is the major source of amnionic fluid after the first trimester?

a. amnionic epithelium
b. fetal urination
c. fetal swallowing
d. fetal inspiration

29–12. What is the most likely cause of increased amnionic fluid in cases of anencephaly?

a. decreased swallowing
b. increased transudation
c. decreased urination
d. increased fetal urine output

29–13. Hydramnios owing to maternal diabetes is most likely the result of which of the following?

a. good glucose control
b. increased fetal urination
c. decreased fetal swallowing
d. osmotic diuresis

29–14. Which of the following is NOT a maternal symptom associated with hydramnios?

a. edema
b. respiratory distress
c. ileus
d. preterm labor

29–15. What is a frequent maternal complication of hydramnios?

a. preeclampsia
b. hypertonic uterine activity
c. placental abruption
d. postterm pregnancy

29–16. How much amniotic fluid should be removed per hour during therapeutic amniocentesis for hydramnios?

a. 100 mL
b. 250 mL
c. 500 mL
d. 1000 mL

29–17. Which drug, when given orally to mothers, may decrease fetal urine output?

a. aspirin
b. cimetidine
c. ranitidine
d. indomethacin

29–18. What is the side effect of using indomethacin for the management of hydramnios?

a. altered neonatal bleeding times
b. maternal nausea and vomiting
c. partial constriction of the fetal ductus arteriosus
d. premature separation of the placenta

29–19. Based on sonographic findings, how is oligohydramnios defined?

a. largest pocket of amniotic fluid <2 cm
b. amniotic fluid index <5 cm
c. AFI <10th percentile
d. none of the above

29–20. What is the most common cause of oligohydramnios?

a. renal anomalies
b. fetal growth retardation
c. twin–twin transfusion
d. premature rupture of fetal membranes

29–21. Which class of drugs is associated with oligohydramnios?

    a. angiotensin-converting enzyme inhibitors

    b. α-adrenergic blockers

    c. calcium-channel blocking agents

    d. β-adrenergic blocking agents

29–22. Of the following, which treatment may increase the amniotic fluid volume?

    a. intravenous saline bolus

    b. decrease salt intake

    c. increased magnesium intake

    d. bromocriptine

29–23. Which of the following findings in the fetus is NOT associated with oligohydramnios?

    a. club foot

    b. dry, leathery, wrinkled skin

    c. decreased subcutaneous tissues

    d. pulmonary hypoplasia

30

Diseases and Abnormalities of the Placenta

30–1. What is the name for incomplete division of the placenta with fetal vessels extending from one lobe to the other?

    a. placenta bipartia

    b. placenta succenturiata

    c. placenta membranacea

    d. fenestrated placenta

30–2. What is the name for small accessory lobes that develop in the fetal membranes?

    a. fenestrated placenta

    b. placenta bipartia

    c. placenta succenturiata

    d. placenta membranacea

30–3. What is the incidence of placenta succenturiata?

    a. 0.3%

    b. 3.0%

    c. 10.0%

    d. 30.0%

30–4. Of the abnormal placentations, which is NOT associated with postpartum hemorrhage?

    a. placenta bipartia

    b. placenta succenturiata

    c. fenestrated placenta

    d. ring-shaped placenta

30–5. Of the abnormal placentas listed, which is associated with fetal growth retardation?

    a. placenta succenturiata

    b. placenta membranacea

    c. fenestrated placenta

    d. ring-shaped placenta

30–6. In which placental type is the chorionic plate smaller than the basal plate?

    a. membranaceous placenta

    b. ring-shaped placenta

    c. extrachorial placenta

    d. fenestrated placenta

30–7. What is the average weight of a normal term placenta?

a. 250 g
b. 500 g
c. 750 g
d. 1000 g

30–8. Retention of normal placenta after delivery is associated with which of the following?

a. placenta previa with next pregnancy
b. placental infarction
c. placental polyps
d. chorioamnionitis with subsequent pregnancy

30–9. Which of the following is the most common placental lesion?

a. previa
b. abruption
c. infarcts
d. deciduitis

30–10. Which of the following are histological features associated with placental infarcts?

a. fibrinoid degeneration of trophoblast; calcification
b. fibrinoid degeneration of trophoblast; plasma cell infiltration
c. fibrinoid degeneration of decidua; calcification
d. fibrinoid degeneration of decidua; plasma cell infiltration

30–11. Which of the following is NOT a morphological indication of aging in a term placenta?

a. syncytial degeneration
b. villous stroma hyalinization
c. clotting beneath the syncytium
d. regeneration of trophoblast

30–12. What is the incidence of placental infarcts in term uncomplicated pregnancies?

a. 10%
b. 25%
c. 50%
d. 67%

30–13. What is the incidence of placental infarcts in pregnancies complicated by severe hypertension?

a. 25%
b. 33%
c. 50%
d. 67%

30–14. At what point in pregnancy do you expect to see calcification in more than half of placentas examined?

a. 21 weeks
b. 25 weeks
c. 29 weeks
d. 33 weeks

30–15. Villous (fetal) artery thrombosis is NOT associated with which of these conditions?

a. diabetes
b. twins
c. maternal antiplatelet antibodies
d. stillbirth

30–16. Striking enlargement of the chorionic villi is associated with which of these conditions?

a. erythroblastosis
b. cytomegalovirus infection
c. syphilis
d. class A diabetes

30–17. In which of the following conditions are cytotrophoblastic cells increased at term?

a. fetal growth retardation
b. diabetes
c. systemic lupus erythematosus
d. hyperthyroidism

30–18. What is the mean length of the normal umbilical cord at term?

a. 25 cm
b. 35 cm
c. 45 cm
d. 55 cm

30–19. Which of the following is NOT increased in pregnancies with long umbilical cords?

a. abruptio placenta
b. uterine inversion
c. true knots
d. chorioamnionitis

30–20. What percentage of infants missing one umbilical artery will have congenital anomalies?

   a. 3
   b. 10
   c. 30
   d. 50

30–21. Which of the following is NOT increased in fetuses with hypercoiled cords?

   a. postterm pregnancy
   b. meconium-stained amniotic fluid
   c. fetal distress
   d. preterm birth

30–22. What is insertion of the cord at the placental margin called?

   a. velamentous insertion
   b. vasa previa
   c. Battledore placenta
   d. true knot

30–23. In what type of placenta do the umbilical vessels separate in the membranes some distance from the placental margin?

   a. velamentous insertion
   b. vasa previa
   c. Battledore placenta
   d. true knot

30–24. Which condition results from active fetal movements?

   a. vasa previa
   b. Battledore placenta
   c. true knots
   d. false knots

30–25. What is the etiology of true knots?

   a. excessive umbilical cord length
   b. active fetus
   c. dizygotic twins
   d. short umbilical cord

30–26. What is the incidence of single-loop nuchal cords?

   a. 0.2%
   b. 2.0%
   c. 20%
   d. 50%

30–27. Which of the following is associated with cord stricture?

   a. focal deficiency of Wharton's jelly
   b. hyperactive fetus during early third trimester
   c. twins
   d. maternal activity

30–28. What is the etiology of true cysts?

   a. intra-amniotic infection
   b. remnants of the allantois
   c. liquefaction of Wharton's jelly
   d. found associated with congenital anomalies

30–29. What is the etiology of false cysts of the umbilical cord?

   a. intra-amniotic infection
   b. remnants of the allantois
   c. liquefaction of Wharton's jelly
   d. found associated with congenital anomalies

30–30. Which of the following is NOT included in the clinical classification of low-risk gestational trophoblastic tumor?

   a. lung metastasis
   b. prior chemotherapy
   c. serum HCG of 36,000 U/mL
   d. symptoms less than 3 months

30–31. What is the incidence of nonmetastatic gestational trophoblastic disease following a partial mole?

   a. 1 to 2%
   b. 4 to 8%
   c. 15 to 20%
   d. 40 to 50%

30–32. What is the etiology of theca-lutein cysts?

   a. abnormal karyotype
   b. increased prolactin receptors
   c. increased follicle-stimulating hormone
   d. increased chorionic gonadotropin

30–33. At what maternal age does the highest frequency of molar pregnancy occur?

   a. 15 to 20 years
   b. 25 to 30 years
   c. 35 to 40 years
   d. >45 years

30–34. What is the most common symptom of molar pregnancy?

a. increased weight gain
b. increased uterine size
c. bleeding
d. increased morning sickness

30–35. What causes the increase in plasma thyroxine in women with molar pregnancies?

a. fetal thyroxine production
b. primarily estrogen-induced increased thyroxine
c. free thyroxine is increased due to human chorionic gonadotropin
d. unknown

30–36. How is the diagnosis of a hydatidiform mole made?

a. x-ray
b. ultrasound
c. computed tomographic pelvimetry
d. magnetic resonance imaging

30–37. What is the treatment of choice for a 16-week-size hydatidiform mole?

a. sharp curettage
b. prostaglandin induction
c. suction evacuation
d. hysterotomy

30–38. In which case below is the incidence of malignant trophoblastic disease increased?

a. partial molar pregnancies
b. advanced maternal age (>40 years)
c. teenager
d. the presence of a 14-cm, theca-lutein cyst

30–39. When used after molar pregnancy, oral contraceptives have been associated with which of the following?

a. more rapid decline in serial chorionic gonadotropin
b. blocking the fall in serial chorionic gonadotropin
c. delaying the decline in serial chorionic gonadotropin
d. no alteration in serial chorionic gonadotropin decline

30–40. What percentage of gestational trophoblastic tumors follow normal pregnancy?

a. 10
b. 25
c. 33
d. 50

30–41. What is the histological diagnostic feature of choriocarcinoma?

a. an increase in cytotrophoblast
b. a decrease in syncytial trophoblast
c. an absent villous pattern
d. an absence of cellular anaplasia

30–42. What is the most common site of metastatic trophoblastic disease?

a. vagina
b. lungs
c. brain
d. ovaries

30–43. Which of the following is characteristic of placental site trophoblastic tumors?

a. predominantly cytotrophoblast
b. predominantly syncytial trophoblast
c. absent villous pattern
d. increased gonadotropin-producing cells

30–44. Which is the drug of choice for persistent gestational trophoblastic disease?

a. doxorubicin (Adriamycin)
b. cisplatin
c. methotrexate
d. actinomycin D

30–45. Which is the therapy of choice for high-risk metastatic disease?

a. etoposide, methotrexate, actinomycin, cyclophosphamide, vinicristine
b. methotrexate alone
c. MAC (methotrexate, actinomycin, and cyclophosphamide)
d. methotrexate and dactinomycin

30–46. Which of the following pregnancy complications may be owing to large chorioangiomas?

a. oligohydramnios
b. polyhydramnios

c. abruption

d. severe hypertension

30–47. In which of the following is embryonic tissue identified?

a. complete molar pregnancy

b. partial molar pregnancy

c. both

d. neither

30–48. Which of the following is characterized by diffuse trophoblastic hyperplasia?

a. complete molar pregnancy

b. partial molar pregnancy

c. both

d. neither

30–49. Which of the following has no villous scalloping?

a. complete molar pregnancy

b. partial molar pregnancy

c. both

d. neither

30–50. Which of the following is characteristic of triploidy 69,XXY?

a. complete molar pregnancy

b. partial molar pregnancy

c. both

d. neither

30–51. In which of the following is choriocarcinoma identified in less than 5 percent of cases?

a. complete molar pregnancy

b. partial molar pregnancy

c. both

d. neither

30–52. Which of the following is characterized by focal hydatidiform swelling?

a. complete molar pregnancy

b. partial molar pregnancy

c. both

d. neither

30–53. Which of the following tumors is likely to metastasize to the placenta?

a. breast cancer

b. melanoma

c. lung cancer

d. endometrial cancer

Common Complications of Pregnancy

31

Hypertensive Disorders in Pregnancy

31–1. Approximately how many women a year die from eclampsia?

   a. 1000
   b. 5000
   c. 10,000
   d. 50,000

31–2. Which of the following is likely to develop true preeclampsia?

   a. a 16-year-old primigravida
   b. a 24-year-old Gr 4, P3
   c. a 25-year-old primigravida
   d. a 35-year-old with essential hypertension

31–3. Which Korotkoff phase sound is used to diagnose pregnancy-induced hypertension?

   a. phase III
   b. phase IV
   c. phase V
   d. phase VI

31–4. In regard to preeclampsia, proteinuria is defined as how much urinary excretion?

   a. >100 mg/24 hr
   b. >200 mg/24 hr
   c. >300 mg/24 hr
   d. >500 mg/24 hr

31–5. Which of the following is NOT diagnostic of severe preeclampsia?

   a. increased serum creatinine
   b. 1+ proteinuria
   c. thrombocytopenia
   d. elevated liver enzymes

31–6. Which of the following is considered an abnormal 24-hour urinary protein?

   a. >300 mg in 24 hr
   b. >1 g in 24 hr
   c. >2 g in 24 hr
   d. >4 g in 24 hr

31–7. With preeclampsia, what is the significance of severe, right upper-quadrant pain?

    a. cholecystitis
    b. pancreatitis
    c. tension on Glisson's capsule
    d. Teitze syndrome

31–8. When is eclampsia least likely to occur?

    a. antepartum
    b. intrapartum
    c. immediately postpartum
    d. after 48 hr postpartum

31–9. How is the pathophysiology of preeclampsia characterized?

    a. vasodilatation
    b. vasospasm
    c. hemodilution
    d. hypervolemia

31–10. Which of the following characterizes normotensive pregnant women?

    a. are refractory to angiotensin II
    b. are sensitive to angiotensin II
    c. react to angiotensin II similar to non-pregnant females
    d. react to angiotensin II similar to males

31–11. What is the incidence of pregnancy-induced hypertension?

    a. <1%
    b. 2 to 3%
    c. 5 to 7%
    d. >10%

31–12. Which of the following is associated with severe preeclampsia?

    a. HLA-DR IgG
    b. molecular variant of angiotensinogen gene
    c. factor V Leiden mutation
    d. renin gene RFLP

31–13. Which of the following is true in preeclamptic women?

    a. Thromboxane is increased.
    b. Prostacyclin is reduced.
    c. Prostaglandin E_2 is decreased.
    d. all of the above

31–14. Low-dose aspirin given to pregnant women causes which of the following?

    a. decreases thromboxane
    b. increases prostacyclin
    c. increases prostaglandin E_2
    d. all of the above

31–15. Hemodynamically in preeclampsia, which of the following is true?

    a. Myocontractility is usually impaired.
    b. Preload is normal or low in the absence of volume expansion.
    c. Hydralazine decreases cardiac output.
    d. As vascular resistance increases, so does cardiac output.

31–16. Which of the following best characterizes the effects of 81 mg of aspirin taken daily?

    a. ↑ thromboxane A_2; ↑ prostacyclin; ↑ prostaglandin E_2
    b. ↑ thromboxane A_2; ↓ prostacyclin; ↑ prostaglandin E_2
    c. ↓ thromboxane A_2; ↓ prostacyclin; ↓ prostaglandin E_2
    d. ↓ thromboxane A_2; ↑ prostacyclin; ↓ prostaglandin E_2

31–17. Which of the following characterizes nitric oxide in hypertension?

    a. increased production
    b. decreased release
    c. decreased production
    d. no change

31–18. Which of the following is true concerning blood volume in eclampsia?

    a. similar to the nonpregnant state
    b. similar to the normal pregnant state
    c. lower than the nonpregnant state
    d. increased compared with the normal pregnant state

31–19. What is the significance of maternal thrombocytopenia in a patient with preeclampsia?

    a. is a fetal indication for cesarean section
    b. indicates severe disease
    c. requires therapy with platelets
    d. is a contraindication to scalp pH determination

31–20. Which of the following is NOT an abnormal erythrocyte finding in severe pregnancy-induced hypertension?

　　a. discocyte
　　b. schizocyte
　　c. spherocytosis
　　d. ecchinocyte

31–21. Which of the following is noted with aldosterone?

　　a. is increased in pregnancy
　　b. is relatively decreased in preeclampsia
　　c. declines as angiotensin II declines
　　d. all of the above

31–22. Which of the following is the characteristic glomerular lesion of preeclampsia?

　　a. endotheliosis
　　b. capillary leaks
　　c. burst cells
　　d. clang cell

31–23. What percentage of women with preeclampsia have CT scan evidence of hepatic hemorrhage?

　　a. <1%
　　b. 2 to 3%
　　c. 5 to 7%
　　d. >10%

31–24. With eclampsia, which of the following is NOT true?

　　a. Cerebral edema is present.
　　b. Electroencephalogram abnormalities are frequent.
　　c. Petechial hemorrhage is common.
　　d. Cerebral blood flow is normal.

31–25. Which of the following is true of blindness in conjunction with severe preeclampsia?

　　a. likely central in origin
　　b. often permanent
　　c. usually unilateral
　　d. common

31–26. What does uterine blood flow in normal-term pregnant women approximate?

　　a. 100 to 200 mL/min
　　b. 200 to 300 mL/min

　　c. 500 to 700 mL/min
　　d. 700 to 900 mL/min

31–27. What is the mean diameter of the spiral arterioles in women with preeclampsia?

　　a. 50 μm
　　b. 100 μm
　　c. 200 μm
　　d. 500 μm

31–28. Which of the following is true of placental blood flow?

　　a. increased by furosemide
　　b. decreased by apresoline
　　c. increased by thiazide diuretics
　　d. increased in patients with preeclampsia

31–29. Of the following, which is NOT considered to be a predisposing factor to preeclampsia?

　　a. family history of preeclampsia
　　b. multiple fetuses
　　c. renal transplantation
　　d. multiparity

31–30. Which of the following is an adverse effect on the fetus when the mother takes thiazide diuretics?

　　a. postterm pregnancy
　　b. congenital malformations
　　c. thrombocytopenia
　　d. microcephalus

31–31. Which of the following is NOT an indication of severe pregnancy-induced hypertension?

　　a. upper abdominal pain
　　b. oliguria
　　c. creatinine 0.6 mg/dL
　　d. fetal growth retardation

31–32. Which of the following is relatively reduced in women with preeclampsia?

　　a. renin
　　b. angiotensin II
　　c. aldosterone
　　d. all of the above

31–33. What is the effect of atrial natriuretic peptide?

    a. increased cardiac output
    b. increased vasospasm
    c. conservation of sodium
    d. conservation of water

31–34. In most women with preeclampsia, how long does it take for proteinuria to resolve?

    a. 2 days
    b. 3 days
    c. 5 days
    d. 7 days

31–35. In women with preeclampsia, what is the cause of acute tubular necrosis?

    a. severe hypertension
    b. fragmentation hemolysis
    c. hemorrhage with inadequate replacement
    d. glomerular capillary endotheliosis

31–36. Which of the following is contraindicated in the treatment of chronic hypertension and pregnancy?

    a. methyldopa
    b. hydralazine
    c. angiotensin-converting enzyme inhibitors
    d. labetolol

31–37. Which of the following is true concerning pregnancy-induced hypertension?

    a. usually resolves within 2 weeks
    b. is not a contraindication to oral contraceptives
    c. postpartum occasionally requires antihypertensive therapy
    d. all of the above

31–38. What plasma magnesium level most often prevents seizures?

    a. 3 to 4 mEq/L
    b. 4 to 7 mEq/L
    c. 7 to 10 mEq/L
    d. over 10 mEq/L

31–39. With a serum creatinine of 1.3 mg/dL, what should be the dose of $MgSO_4$?

    a. increased
    b. kept the same
    c. reduced by half
    d. discontinued

31–40. How is magnesium excreted?

    a. lungs
    b. liver
    c. kidney
    d. gastrointestinal tract

31–41. At what serum level of magnesium do patellar reflexes disappear?

    a. 6 mEq/L
    b. 8 mEq/L
    c. 10 mEq/L
    d. 12 mEq/L

31–42. How is magnesium toxicity treated?

    a. calcium gluconate 1 g intravenously
    b. calcium gluconate orally
    c. calcium gluconate and discontinue magnesium
    d. dialysis

31–43. In severe preeclampsia with pulmonary edema, what immediate treatment should be given?

    a. furosemide intravenously
    b. digoxin
    c. hydrochlorothiazide
    d. fluid restriction

31–44. What is the recurrence rate of eclampsia?

    a. 2%
    b. 8%
    c. 17%
    d. 25%

31–45. Following preeclampsia–eclampsia, what is the incidence of chronic hypertension?

    a. less than in the general population
    b. the same as in the general population
    c. double that in the general population
    d. four times that in the general population

32

Obstetrical Hemorrhage

32–1. What is the incidence of direct obstetrical death owing to hemorrhage?

    a. 1 to 5% of cases
    b. 10 to 15% of cases
    c. 25 to 30% of cases
    d. 50 to 65% of cases

32–2. Which of the following is characteristic of midtrimester bleeding?

    a. little consequence
    b. related to early effacement and tearing of small vessels
    c. 25 percent of the time a previa or an abruption will be found
    d. requires hospitalization

32–3. Which of the following is most commonly associated with placental abruption?

    a. trauma
    b. short umbilical cord
    c. folic acid deficiency
    d. hypertension

32–4. What is the frequency of placental abruption?

    a. 1 in 50
    b. 1 in 100
    c. 1 in 150
    d. 1 in 200

32–5. What is the incidence of abruption severe enough to kill the fetus?

    a. 1 in 200
    b. 1 in 420
    c. 1 in 830
    d. 1 in 1100

32–6. What is the approximate risk of recurrent abruption with a subsequent pregnancy?

    a. 0.4%
    b. 12%
    c. 20%
    d. 33%

32–7. What is the most common presenting sign in women with abruptio placenta?

    a. preterm labor
    b. uterine tenderness
    c. back pain
    d. bleeding

32–8. What percentage of the total pregnant blood volume is lost with an abruption severe enough to cause fetal demise?

    a. 5
    b. 10
    c. 25
    d. 50 or greater

32– 9. Which compound is responsible for lysing fibrin?

    a. thromboplastin
    b. plasmin
    c. prostacyclin
    d. factor III

32–10. How can acute tubular necrosis following abruption be prevented?

    a. cesarean section
    b. volume replacement
    c. furosemide
    d. Swan-Ganz catheter

32–11. Which of the following is characteristic of a Couvelaire uterus?

   a. need for hysterectomy
   b. contracts well with stimulation
   c. results from excessive oxytocin
   d. requires fibrinogen therapy

32–12. Which of the following is the most ideal method of delivery for severe abruption with fetal demise?

   a. vaginal delivery
   b. immediate cesarean section
   c. cesarean section after blood replacement
   d. cesarean section after 5 units of cryoprecipitate

32–13. What is the baseline intra-amniotic pressure with extensive placental abruption?

   a. 0
   b. 5 to 10 mm Hg
   c. 15 to 50 mm Hg
   d. >100 mm Hg

32–14. What percentage of patients develop hypofibrinogenemia with a severe abruption and a dead fetus?

   a. 10
   b. 30
   c. 50
   d. 65

32–15. With a severe abruption and associated hypofibrinogenemia, which of the following is indicated prior to surgery?

   a. heparin
   b. low-molecular-weight heparin
   c. epsilon-aminocaproic acid
   d. cryoprecipitate

32–16. What is the incidence of placenta previa at term?

   a. 1 in 50 pregnancies
   b. 1 in 200 pregnancies
   c. 1 in 400 pregnancies
   d. 1 in 800 pregnancies

32–17. Which of the following is least likely to result in a patient having placenta previa?

   a. primiparity
   b. previous cesarean section
   c. multiparity
   d. advancing maternal age

32–18. What is the incidence of previa in a woman with three previous cesarean sections?

   a. 0.5%
   b. 1.9%
   c. 3.1%
   d. 4.1%

32–19. What is the most common characteristic sign or symptom in women with placenta previa?

   a. abnormal fetal heart rate tracing
   b. painful bleeding
   c. painless bleeding
   d. coagulopathy

32–19. What is the most common method for diagnosis of placenta previa?

   a. abdominal x-ray
   b. arteriography
   c. ultrasound
   d. computed tomographic scanning

32–21. Which of the following may be of benefit in a woman with a dead fetus who develops coagulopathy?

   a. heparin
   b. cryoprecipitate
   c. epsilon-aminocaproic acid
   d. factor VIII concentrates

32–22. Which of the following is the most common cause of postpartum hemorrhage mandating hysterectomy?

   a. previa
   b. atony
   c. irreparable tears
   d. placental accreta

32–23. Assuming blood loss is 1000 mL, how is late postpartum hemorrhage defined?

   a. 1 hr
   b. 2 hr
   c. 8 hr
   d. 24 hr

32–24. What are the two most common causes of hemorrhage?

    a. uterine atony and retained placenta
    b. retained placenta and lacerations
    c. lacerations and uterine atony
    d. chorioamnionitis and retained placenta

32–25. Which of the following is NOT a predisposing factor to postpartum hemorrhage?

    a. prolonged labor
    b. term twins
    c. rapid labor
    d. patient with 1500-g infant

32–26. Given a postpartum hemorrhage, which of the following patients would be in greatest danger?

    a. height 5'0" ~100 lb
    b. height 5'0" ~100 lb with preeclampsia
    c. height 5'8" ~180 lb
    d. height 5'8" ~180 lb with preeclampsia

32–27. Bright red bleeding that continues even in the presence of a firmly contracted uterus is most likely due to which of the following?

    a. thrombocytopenia
    b. retained placenta
    c. lacerations
    d. ruptured uterus

32–28. Which of the following is NOT a characteristic of Sheehan syndrome?

    a. profuse lactation
    b. amenorrhea
    c. loss of axillary and pubic hair
    d. adrenal insufficiency

32–29. Following delivery of the placenta, which of the following is contraindicated?

    a. methergine 0.2 mg intramuscularly
    b. 20 U of oxytocin in 1000 mL Ringer's lactate solution
    c. 20 U of oxytocin intravenous bolus
    d. uterine massage

32–30. Oxytocin may cause which of the following?

    a. hypotension and cardiac arrhythmias
    b. hypertension and myometrial contractions

    c. hypotension and myometrial contractions
    d. hypertension and cardiac arrhythmias

32–31. Intramuscular prostaglandin is used to treat hemorrhage owing to atony. What is the prostaglandin dosage?

    a. 15-methyl $F_{2\alpha}$ 1 g
    b. 15-methyl $F_{2\alpha}$ .25 mg
    c. 15-methyl E_2 1 g
    d. 15-methyl E_2 .25 mg

32–32. When using carboprost, what happens to the PO_2?

    a. rises
    b. decreases
    c. remains unchanged
    d. drops initially then levels off (asthma to improve)

32–33. Which of the following is characteristic of placenta accreta?

    a. Nitabuch's layer is absent.
    b. Villi invade the myometrium.
    c. Villi penetrate the myometrium.
    d. Villi invade the parietal peritoneum.

32–34. Which of the following is a microscopic feature of placenta accreta?

    a. cicatrix
    b. absence of Nitabuch layer
    c. hypertrophy of the decidua
    d. trophoblastic proliferation

32–35. How should placenta accreta be best managed?

    a. cutting the cord and using oxytocin
    b. observation
    c. hysterectomy
    d. hypogastric artery ligation

32–36. A woman with which of the following is least likely to have a placenta accreta?

    a. previous cesarean section
    b. previous metroplasty
    c. four previous curettages
    d. gravida 1, para 0

32–37. What anesthetic agent is most ideal for replacing an inverted uterus?

    a. spinal analgesia
    b. thiopental
    c. succinylcholine
    d. halothane

32–38. A postpartum vulvar hematoma is limited superiorly by which of the following?

    a. Colle's fascia
    b. round ligament
    c. levator ani
    d. the peritoneum

32–39. Which artery is most often associated with vulvar hematomas?

    a. uterine
    b. cervical
    c. femoral
    d. pudendal

32–40. What is the most common presenting complaint with vulvar hematomas?

    a. excruciating pain
    b. hemorrhage
    c. constipation
    d. urinary retention

32–41. What is the approximate incidence of uterine rupture in an unscarred uterus?

    a. 1 in 200
    b. 1 in 2000
    c. 1 in 20,000
    d. 1 in 200,000

32–42. What is the most common cause of uterine rupture?

    a. previous uterine perforation
    b. excessive oxytocin
    c. manual manipulation (i.e., internal version)
    d. separation of a previous cesarean section scar

32–43. What proportion of classical scar ruptures occur before labor?

    a. all
    b. one-half
    c. one-third
    d. one-fourth

32–44. What is the incidence of separation of the previous low transverse uterine scar during trial of labor?

    a. 1 in 20
    b. 1 in 100
    c. 1 in 200
    d. 1 in 500

32–45. What is the maternal febrile morbidity in a woman undergoing a trial of labor compared to elective repeat cesarean section?

    a. slightly increased
    b. markedly increased
    c. the same
    d. decreased by one-half

32–46. Which of the following is NOT a major risk factor for rupture of the unscarred uterus?

    a. oxytocin infusion
    b. parity
    c. prostaglandin E_2 gel
    d. age less than 15 years

32–47. Which of the following is considered a "classical" finding in uterine rupture?

    a. increased vaginal bleeding
    b. sharp, shooting pain
    c. sudden increase in uterine contraction
    d. sudden loss of fetal heart tones

32–48. What is the incidence of fetal mortality in the presence of uterine rupture?

    a. 5 to 10%
    b. 25 to 30%
    c. 50 to 75%
    d. >90%

32–49. Where is the ureter found with respect to the location of the ligature in internal iliac artery ligation?

    a. superiorly
    b. inferiorly
    c. medially
    d. laterally

32–50. What is the important mechanism in the efficacy of internal iliac artery ligation?

    a. ischemia
    b. reduction in pulse/pressure
    c. block of collateral circulation
    d. all of the above

32–51. What is the origin of the internal iliac artery?

    a. ovarian
    b. aorta
    c. common iliac
    d. external iliac

32–52. Urinary incontinence may develop secondary to injury of which muscle during vaginal delivery?

    a. iliococcygeus muscle
    b. external sphincter ani
    c. puborectalis
    d. pubococcygeus

33

Hypovolemic Shock and Disseminated Intravascular Coagulation

33–1. In general, what is the average decrease in hematocrit postpartum for women delivering vaginally?

    a. <1%
    b. 2 to 3%
    c. 5 to 8%
    d. >10%

33–2. What is the average decrease in hematocrit after a cesarean delivery?

    a. <1%
    b. 3 to 5%
    c. 8 to 10%
    d. >15%

33–3. Which of the following is NOT characteristic of early hypovolemic shock?

    a. decreased mean arterial pressure
    b. decreased stroke volume
    c. increased arteriovenous oxygen content difference
    d. increased central venous pressure

33–4. Which of the following is activated and responsible for leukocyte–endothelial cell interaction?

    a. CD 18 locus
    b. ΔDF_{508}
    c. platelet aggregation
    d. cytochrome P450

33–5. During shock, at what level should urine blood flow be maintained to prevent renal tubular acidosis?

    a. 0.1 mL/kg
    b. 1.0 mL/kg
    c. 5.0 mL/kg
    d. 10.0 mL/kg

33–6. At what hemoglobin concentration does cardiac output substantively increase?

    a. 5.0 g/dL
    b. 7.0 g/dL
    c. 8.5 g/dL
    d. 17.0 g/dL

33–7. How much fibrinogen is supplied in one unit of fresh frozen plasma?

    a. 50 mg
    b. 100 mg
    c. 150 mg
    d. 200 mg

33–8. By how much will the hematocrit increase after one unit of whole blood?

    a. <0.5 vol%
    b. 1 to 2 vol%
    c. 3 to 5 vol%
    d. 6 to 8 vol%

33–9. What is the most frequent coagulation defect found in women with blood loss and multiple transfusions?

    a. thrombocytopenia
    b. prolonged PT
    c. prolonged whole bleeding time
    d. AT-III deficiency

33–10. What is the hematocrit in a unit of packed red cells?

    a. 35 vol%
    b. 45 to 50 vol%
    c. 60 to 70 vol%
    d. 80 to 90 vol%

33–11. Which of the following factors is NOT a component of cryoprecipitate?

    a. factor VIII:C
    b. fetal fibronectin
    c. factor VIII von Willebrand
    d. fibrinogen

33–12. What is the risk of HIV infection after one unit of blood?

    a. 1 in 150,000
    b. 1 in 300,000
    c. 1 in 600,000
    d. 1 in 900,000

33–13. What is the risk of post-transfusion hepatitis C?

    a. 1 in 3000
    b. 1 in 6000

    c. 1 in 12,000
    d. 1 in 25,000

33–14. Which of the following factors is NOT increased during normal pregnancy?

    a. fibrinogen
    b. VII
    c. VIII
    d. XI

33–15. At what fibrinogen level can you expect to see lack of clinical coagulation?

    a. 25 mg/dL
    b. 50 mg/dL
    c. 100 mg/dL
    d. 150 mg/dL

33–16. What is the most common cause of severe consumptive coagulopathy in pregnancy?

    a. fetal death
    b. placenta previa
    c. placental abruption
    d. sepsis

33–17. Which of the following is NOT characteristic of amniotic fluid embolism?

    a. chest pain
    b. hypotension
    c. hypoxia
    d. consumptive coagulopathy

33–18. Which of the following is characteristic of the secondary phase of amniotic fluid embolism?

    a. pulmonary hypertension
    b. decreased systemic vascular resistance
    c. decreased left ventricular stroke index
    d. lung injury and coagulopathy

33–19. By what mechanism does endotoxin (lipopolysaccharide) activate the extrinsic clotting scheme?

    a. TNF-induced tissue factor expression
    b. blocks thrombotic activity
    c. increases plasmin activity
    d. inhibits thromboplastin

34

Preterm Birth

34-1. Where does the United States rank in infant mortality?

  a. 1st
  b. 11th
  c. 22nd
  d. 44th

34-2. What is the World Health Organization definition of a premature infant?

  a. <2500 g
  b. 38 weeks or less
  c. 37 weeks or less
  d. 36 weeks or less

34-3. What is the definition of an extremely low-birth-weight infant?

  a. <2500 g
  b. <1500 g
  c. <1000 g
  d. <500 g

34-4. In general, at what gestational age and weight are the majority of obstetricians willing to perform a cesarean section for a nonreassuring fetal heart rate pattern?

  a. 24 weeks and 500 g
  b. 24 weeks and 700 g
  c. 26 weeks or 500 g
  d. 26 weeks or 700 g

34-5. At what gestational age does the incidence of complications due to prematurity equal that of term infants?

  a. 25 to 26 weeks
  b. 28 to 30 weeks
  c. 32 to 34 weeks
  d. 36 weeks or more

34-6. What is the least common cause of preterm labor?

  a. rupture of the membranes
  b. idiopathic preterm labor
  c. maternal complication
  d. incompetent cervix

34-7. Which of the following products is NOT found in the amniotic fluid of women with infection associated with preterm labor?

  a. thromboxane
  b. lipopolysaccharide
  c. interleukin-6
  d. tumor necrosis factor

34-8. Which of the following is the most specific test of amniotic fluid to exclude intra-amniotic infection?

  a. glucose
  b. interleukin-6
  c. white blood cell count
  d. gram stain

34-9. Which of these tests is most sensitive?

  a. glucose
  b. interleukin-6
  c. white blood cell count
  d. gram stain

34-10. Which of the following vaginal infections is positively associated with preterm birth?

  a. bacterial vaginosis
  b. trichomonal vaginalis
  c. candida vaginalis
  d. herpes simplex infections

34–11. Which of the following preterm birth-risk scoring systems is universally beneficial?

    a. Papiernik's
    b. Creasy's
    c. MacDonald's
    d. none

34–12. Of the following, which statement is NOT true concerning fetal fibronectin?

    a. It is a glycoprotein.
    b. A positive test correlates closely with preterm birth.
    c. A negative test suggests that preterm labor will not ensue.
    d. It is produced by amnion cells only.

34–13. Which of the following best describes home uterine activity monitoring?

    a. It is investigational.
    b. It is "standard of care."
    c. It delays preterm delivery.
    d. It is approved by ACOG.

34–14. How is preterm labor defined?

    a. regular uterine contractions 5 to 8 min apart
    b. progressive change in the cervix
    c. dilatation to 2 cm or more or 80 percent or more effacement
    d. all of the above

34–15. When using sonography to measure cervical length in women with preterm labor, what is the critical measurement below which all women delivered preterm?

    a. 2 cm
    b. 3 cm
    c. 4 cm
    d. 5 cm

34–16. Which of the following is true for empirical cesarean section for a preterm fetus?

    a. has no scientific merit
    b. results in lower morbidity
    c. results in lower mortality
    d. has decreased in the last 15 years

34–17. With preterm rupture of membranes, in what percentage of cases will delivery occur after 48 hours?

    a. 2
    b. 7

    c. 25
    d. 50

34–18. What is the preferred management of preterm rupture of membranes?

    a. antibiotics
    b. tocolytics
    c. steroids
    d. expectant

34–19. What is the threshold gestational age for lung hypoplasia if the membranes rupture prematurely?

    a. 17 weeks
    b. 20 weeks
    c. 23 weeks
    d. 28 weeks

34–20. Which is true concerning the use of glucocorticoids to promote fetal pulmonary maturation?

    a. results in decreased neonatal mortality
    b. results in decreased respiratory distress syndrome
    c. preferentially benefits the male fetus
    d. is standard therapy since the NIH Consensus Conference

34–21. Which of the following is a maternal effect of ritodrine?

    a. hypoglycemia
    b. hypokalemia
    c. bradycardia
    d. hypertension

34–22. What is the mechanism of action of β-adrenergic agents?

    a. blocks thymidine kinase
    b. activates adenylcyclase
    c. blocks conversion of ATP to cyclic AMP
    d. increases intracellular calcium

34–23. What is the proposed mechanism of action for magnesium sulfate when used for tocolysis?

    a. blocks cAMP
    b. increases intracellular calcium
    c. acts as a calcium antagonist
    d. stimulates β receptors

34–24. Which of the following is NOT true concerning indomethacin?

  a. is used to treat preterm labor
  b. is a prostaglandin synthetase inhibitor
  c. may cause premature closure of the fetal ductus arteriosus
  d. decreases neonatal intracranial hemorrhage

34–25. Which tocolytic agent enhances the toxicity of magnesium to produce neuromuscular blockade?

  a. nifedipine
  b. ritodrine
  c. indomethacin
  d. ethanol

35

Postterm Pregnancy

35–1. How is postterm pregnancy defined?

  a. beyond 37 weeks
  b. beyond 40 weeks
  c. beyond 42 weeks
  d. beyond 44 weeks

35–2. In days, how is a postterm pregnancy defined?

  a. >280 days
  b. >287 days
  c. >294 days
  d. >300 days

35–3. What happens to perinatal mortality after 42 weeks' gestation?

  a. no change
  b. decreases
  c. increases slightly
  d. increases significantly

35–4. Which of the following is characteristic of placental sulfatase deficiency?

  a. associated with preterm labor
  b. is a sex-linked recessive trait
  c. is associated with high urinary estriols
  d. all of the above

35–5. What is the incidence of neonatal seizures in a postterm fetus?

  a. 0.9 per 1000
  b. 1.8 per 1000
  c. 3.6 per 1000
  d. 5.4 per 1000

35–6. Which of the following is true concerning postterm fetal jeopardy?

  a. related to placental insufficiency
  b. related to cord compression with oligohydramnios
  c. an indication for cesarean section
  d. manifested by late deceleration

35–7. Which hormone is secreted in insufficient amounts in pregnancies complicated by anencephaly?

  a. DHEA
  b. DHEA-sulfate
  c. prostaglandin $F_{2\alpha}$
  d. prostaglandin

35–8. What is the incidence of postterm pregnancy in the United States?

    a. 1%
    b. 5 to 6%
    c. 11%
    d. 20%

35–9. Which of the following is NOT a description associated with the postmature infant?

    a. smooth skinned
    b. patchy peeling skin
    c. long, thin body
    d. worried looking fascies

35–10. How are small-for-gestational-age infants defined?

    a. below 2500 g
    b. below 2000 g
    c. below the 10th percentile
    d. below the 20th percentile

35–11. In a woman with a favorable cervix and an estimated fetal weight of 3850 g, what is the appropriate management at a certain 42 weeks' gestation?

    a. expectant management
    b. start fetal surveillance
    c. induce labor
    d. schedule cesarean section

35–12. In a woman with an unfavorable cervix and an estimated fetal weight of 3800 g, what is the appropriate management at a certain 42 weeks' gestation?

    a. labor induction
    b. cesarean section
    c. fetal surveillance plus hospitalization
    d. cervical ripening

35–13. When is the mean daily weight gain of the fetus in utero at its greatest?

    a. 20 weeks
    b. 26 weeks
    c. 30 weeks
    d. 37 weeks

36

Fetal Growth Restriction

36–1. What is the incidence of fetal growth restriction?

    a. <1%
    b. 3 to 10%
    c. 15 to 20%
    d. ~25%

36–2. How are small-for-gestational-age infants defined?

    a. below 2500 g
    b. below 2000 g
    c. below the 10th percentile
    d. below the 20th percentile

36–3. Which of the following is NOT a determinant of infants' birthweight?

    a. ethnicity
    b. parity
    c. maternal weight
    d. 30-lb maternal weight gain during pregnancy

36–4. Which of the following is NOT associated with fetal growth restriction?

    a. birth asphyxia
    b. sepsis
    c. hypoglycemia
    d. hypothermia

36–5. What is characteristic of the first phase of fetal growth?

    a. cellular death
    b. cellular swelling
    c. cellular hyperplasia
    d. cellular hypertrophy

36–6. How is symmetrical growth restriction characterized?

    a. reduction in head size
    b. reduction in body size
    c. reduction in both body and head size
    d. reduction in body and femur length

36–7. What is the brain to liver weight ratio in a severely growth restricted infant?

    a. 1 to 2
    b. 2 to 1
    c. 3 to 1
    d. 5 to 1

36–8. Which of the following is NOT a risk factor for severe fetal growth restriction?

    a. maternal weight less than 100 lb
    b. fetal infections
    c. trisomy 21
    d. smoking

36–9. Which of the following chromosomal disorders is NOT associated with fetal growth restriction?

    a. 45,X
    b. trisomy 18
    c. trisomy 13
    d. fetal growth restriction with all of the above

36–10. Which trisomy is responsible for confirmed placental mosaicism and many cases of previously unexplained fetal growth restriction?

    a. 13
    b. 16
    c. 18
    d. 21

36–11. What is the incidence of fetal alcohol syndrome in women who drink three drinks per day during pregnancy?

    a. <1%
    b. 3 to 5%
    c. 10%
    d. >20%

36–12. Which of the following compounds is elevated in the plasma of growth-restricted fetuses?

    a. prostacyclin
    b. adenosine
    c. interleukin-1
    d. epidermal growth factor

36–13. Which of the following ultrasound measurements is the most reliable index of fetal size?

    a. biparietal diameter
    b. abdominal circumference
    c. femur length
    d. intrathoracic ratio

36–14. Which sonographic measurement in a growth-restricted fetus correlates best with significant perinatal mortality?

    a. biparietal diameter
    b. abdominal circumference
    c. femur length
    d. oligohydramnios

36–15. Which test of fetal well-being correlates with fetal metabolic acidosis at birth?

    a. reactive nonstress test
    b. negative contraction stress test
    c. biophysical profile of 8/10
    d. reversed end-diastolic umbilical artery velocimetry

36–16. Which of the following exemplifies symmetrical growth restriction?

   a. congenital rubella syndrome
   b. hypertension
   c. advanced diabetes
   d. all of the above

36–17. Which of the following is NOT associated with fetal growth restriction?

   a. toxoplasmosis infection
   b. cytomegalovirus infection
   c. congenital rubella
   d. spina bifida

37

Macrosomia

37–1. How is macrosomia defined?

   a. birthweight > 4000 g
   b. birthweight > 4100 g
   c. birthweight > 4500 g
   d. birthweight > 5000 g

37–2. What is the ponderal index?

   a. body weight $\times 50 \div \text{length}^2$
   b. body weight $\times 100 \div \text{length}^2$
   c. body weight $\times 100 \div \text{length}^3$
   d. newborn weight $\div$ length + weight @ 50%

37–3. Which of the following is NOT a risk factor for macrosomia?

   a. diabetes
   b. female fetus
   c. maternal obesity
   d. gestational age > 42 weeks

37–4. What is the best way to estimate fetal size (accurately)?

   a. ultrasound (BPD FL AC = EFW)
   b. x-ray pelvimetry
   c. Leopold's maneuvers
   d. not possible

37–5. Which of the following is NOT a risk of macrosomia?

   a. intraventricular hemorrhage
   b. brachial plexus injury
   c. shoulder dystocia
   d. cephalopelvic disproportion

37–6. At what birthweight is a primary cesarean section justified?

   a. >4000 g
   b. >4250 g
   c. >4500 g
   d. not justified on estimated weight alone

38

Multifetal Pregnancy

38–1. What percentage of twins are monozygous?

    a. 10
    b. 25
    c. 33
    d. 50

38–2. In monozygotic twins, which of the following is true of dichorionic diamnionic membranes?

    a. do not occur
    b. occur if division is prior to 72 hours after fertilization
    c. single placenta almost always noted
    d. division after 72 hours of fertilization

38–3. What is the incidence of monozygotic twins?

    a. 1 in 250
    b. dependent on race
    c. dependent on age
    d. dependent on parity

38–4. Which of the following is true for a chimera?

    a. individual with multiple phenotypes
    b. individual with a mixture of genotypes
    c. involves triple fertilization
    d. is a consequence of nondisjunction

38–5. Which of the following is true concerning the incidence of twins?

    a. most common in the black race
    b. most common in the oriental race
    c. most common in the white race
    d. equal in all races

38–6. What is the association of ovulation induction for infertility with multiple births?

    a. decreases multiple pregnancies
    b. increases multiple pregnancies

    c. increases only dizygotic twins
    d. does not effect the incidence of twins

38–7. Which of the following is true concerning monochorionic diamnionic membranes?

    a. result from monozygosity
    b. result from dizygosity
    c. do not reveal zygosity
    d. none of the above

38–8. Which of the following ultrasound characteristics is an indication of monochorionic twins?

    a. same gender
    b. dividing membrane thickness 1 mm
    c. two placentas
    d. concordancy

38–9. Which is true of preterm twins compared with preterm singletons?

    a. have a greater incidence of cerebral palsy
    b. have a greater incidence of microcephaly
    c. have a greater incidence of encephalomalacia
    d. all of the above

38–10. Which of the following is suggestive of dichorionic diamnionic twin pregnancy?

    a. lack of discordance
    b. sonographic measurement of the dividing membranes greater than 2 mm
    c. two separate placentae
    d. none of the above

38–11. Which of the following is true concerning an abdominal x-ray to diagnose twins?

    a. needs to be done after 18 weeks if indicated
    b. is probably inferior to sonography
    c. may be falsely negative
    d. all of the above

38–12. What is the best management at 32 weeks' gestation when one twin is noted to have died in utero?

a. immediate oxytocin induction of labor
b. immediate delivery by cesarean section
c. observation
d. heparin immediately to prevent coagulopathy

38–13. What is the mean increase in blood volume in twin gestation?

a. 10 to 20%
b. 40 to 50%
c. 50 to 60%
d. 70 to 80%

38–14. What is the average blood loss for twin gestation?

a. ~250 mL
b. 500 mL
c. 750 mL
d. 1000 mL

38–15. What is the incidence of major malformations in twin gestations?

a. <1%
b. 2%
c. 4%
d. 8%

38–16. What is the mean duration of gestation for twins?

a. 33 weeks
b. 35 weeks
c. 37 weeks
d. 39 weeks

38–17. Comparing twins with singletons, which of the following is NOT true?

a. Perinatal mortality is increased.
b. Chromosomal abnormalities are increased.
c. Cerebral palsy is increased.
d. Intelligence is less.

38–18. Which of the following is true concerning superfecundation?

a. probably does not occur
b. requires fertilization of 2 ova at different coital acts

c. requires conception of twins with an interval between conception as long as one menstrual cycle
d. results in mosaicism

38–19. With twins, which of the following is NOT true?

a. Pregnancy hypervolemia approximates 50 to 60%.
b. Cardiac output is increased.
c. Pulse rate is decreased.
d. Stroke volume is increased.

38–20. How is discordance in twins best measured?

a. biparietal diameter
b. abdominal circumference
c. femur length
d. crown-rump length

38–21. Which of the following is NOT a specific complication of monoamnionic twins?

a. cord entanglement
b. discordancy
c. conjoined twins
d. preterm labor

38–22. Which of the following is the most common type of conjoined twins?

a. thoracopagus
b. craniopagus
c. ischiopagus
d. pyopagus

38–23. Which of the following may be involved in the pathophysiology of twin–twin transfusion?

a. multiple superficial vascular anastomoses
b. solitary deep arteriovenous channels
c. venous-venous connection
d. arterial-arterial connection

38–24. Which of the following is NOT a diagnostic criteria for twin–twin transfusion?

a. hemoglobin differences > 5g/dL
b. birthweight differences > 20%
c. oligohydramnios in large twin
d. placental vascular connection

38–25. When twin discordancy exceeds 30 percent, which of the following is true?

    a. increased neonatal deaths
    b. fewer congenital anomalies
    c. less growth restriction
    d. increase in fetal deaths

38–26. What is the daily folic acid requirement or recommendation for twin pregnancy?

    a. 0.1 mg
    b. 0.4 mg
    c. 1 mg
    d. 4 mg

38–27. Which of the following is true concerning antenatal fetal testing in twins?

    a. The best test is an NST.
    b. Antepartum death rates are not different.
    c. Twice weekly biophysical profiles are best.
    d. Doppler velocimetry is the ideal test.

38–28. What is the best prophylactic way to prevent preterm delivery in twins?

    a. bedrest
    b. β-mimetics
    c. cervical cerclage
    d. hospitalization for complications

38–29. What is the most common intrapartum presentation for twins?

    a. cephalic–cephalic
    b. cephalic–breech
    c. breech–breech
    d. breech–cephalic

38–30. Interlocking twins is associated with which of the following presentations?

    a. cephalic–cephalic
    b. cephalic–breech
    c. breech–breech
    d. breech–cephalic

Fetal Abnormalities: Inherited and Acquired Disorders

39

Genetics

39–1. What percentage of newborns have a recognizable birth defect?

    a. <1
    b. 3 to 5
    c. 7 to 8
    d. 10

39–2. Which of the following etiological categories accounts for the majority of fetal anomalies?

    a. chromosomal and single-gene defects
    b. maternal diseases (diabetes, alcohol, etc.)
    c. drugs and medications
    d. multifactorial or unknown

39–3. What is the approximate incidence of chromosomal abnormalities in live-born infants?

    a. 1 in 25
    b. 1 in 75
    c. 1 in 150
    d. 1 in 350

39–4. What is the frequency of chromosomal abnormalities among stillbirths and neonatal deaths?

    a. <1%
    b. 3%
    c. 6 to 7%
    d. 15 to 20%

39–5. What is the most common chromosomal abnormality in early spontaneous abortions?

    a. 45,X
    b. 47,XXY
    c. 47,XXX
    d. trisomy 21

39–6. Which of the following is NOT a characteristic finding in newborns with Down syndrome?

    a. large head
    b. flattened occiput
    c. upslanting palpebral fissures
    d. clinodactyly

39–7. What is the recurrence risk of trisomy 21 in the subsequent children of young mothers?

    a. 1 to 2%
    b. 5%
    c. 12%
    d. 25%

39–8. What is the approximate risk of trisomy 21 in a 20-year-old woman?

    a. 1 in 70
    b. 1 in 150
    c. 1 in 500
    d. 1 in 1400

39–9. What is the approximate risk of trisomy 21 in a 40-year-old woman?

    a. 1 in 70
    b. 1 in 150
    c. 1 in 500
    d. 1 in 1200

39–10. What percentage of Down syndrome pregnancies in women 35 years and older will be lost between 10 weeks (time of CVS) and 16 weeks (time of amniocentesis)?

    a. <5%
    b. 12%
    c. 32%
    d. 53%

39–11. Which of the following types of genetic disease is related to paternal age?

    a. trisomies
    b. multifactorial diseases
    c. translocations
    d. autosomal dominant disease

39–12. What deletion is responsible for the cri du chat syndrome?

    a. del (4p)
    b. del (5p)
    c. del (21p)
    d. del (Xp)

39–13. Which of the following chromosomes is generally NOT involved in Robertsonian translocation?

    a. 1
    b. 13

    c. 14
    d. 21

39–14. What is the approximate recurrence risk of a translocation Down syndrome that occurred spontaneously (i.e., neither parent is a carrier)?

    a. 1%
    b. 5%
    c. 25%
    d. 50%

39–15. In the event of a 21/21 translocation in one parent, what is the chance of having a child with Down syndrome?

    a. 1 to 2%
    b. 5%
    c. 50%
    d. 100%

39–16. Approximately what percentage of couples with recurrent pregnancy loss will have either a balanced Robertsonian or reciprocal translocation?

    a. 2
    b. 10
    c. 25
    d. 50

39–17. Which of the following traits is usually not found in offspring with 45,X monosomy?

    a. short
    b. webbing of the neck
    c. coarctation of the aorta
    d. mental retardation

39–18. Which of the following usually is NOT found in offspring with 47,XXY?

    a. truncal obesity
    b. gynecomastia
    c. decreased serum gonadotropin levels
    d. azoospermia

39–19. Which of the following traits is NOT characteristic of offspring with an extra Y chromosome (47,XYY)?

    a. tall
    b. severe acne
    c. learning disabilities
    d. severe mental retardation

39–20. Which of the following is NOT a characteristic of autosomal dominant inheritance?

  a. a single copy of the mutant gene present
  b. horizontal transmission
  c. no skipped generations
  d. 50 percent chance of transmission to the offspring

39–21. What is the incidence of newborns with a phenotypic abnormality secondary to a Mendelian disorder?

  a. 1 per 100
  b. 1 per 1000
  c. 1 per 10,000
  d. 1 per 50,000

39–22. Which of the following conditions is NOT inherited in an autosomal dominant fashion?

  a. achondroplasia
  b. adult polycystic kidney disease
  c. Marfan syndrome
  d. cystic fibrosis

39–23. What is the mechanism by which the expression of a particular disease is dependent on whether the mutant gene was of paternal or maternal origin?

  a. penetrance
  b. imprinting
  c. uniparental disomy
  d. anticipation

39–24. What is the mechanism by which some autosomal dominant diseases appear to occur at earlier ages with subsequent generations?

  a. penetrance
  b. imprinting
  c. variable expressivity
  d. anticipation

39–25. What is the mechanism by which both members of one pair of chromosomes are inherited from the same parent?

  a. imprinting
  b. variable expressivity
  c. uniparental disomy
  d. anticipation

39–26. Which of the following is NOT an autosomal recessive disease?

  a. Tay-Sachs disease
  b. congenital adrenal hyperplasia
  c. myotonic dystrophy
  d. sickle cell disease

39–27. Which of the following is an X-linked disease?

  a. Von Willebrand disease
  b. neurofibromatosis
  c. Hunter syndrome
  d. Tay-Sachs disease

39–28. What is the risk of having anomalous children resulting from incest (brother–sister or parent–child)?

  a. 5%
  b. 10%
  c. 25%
  d. 50%

39–29. What proportion of genes do first cousins share?

  a. 1/2
  b. 1/4
  c. 1/8
  d. 1/16

39–30. Mothers with PKU are at increased risk of having a child with which of the following disorders?

  a. hydrocephaly
  b. spina bifida
  c. skeletal dysplasia
  d. mental retardation

39–31. Which of the following is an example of an X-linked dominant disorder?

  a. vitamin D-resistant rickets
  b. hemophilia A
  c. hemophilia B
  d. muscular dystrophy

39–32. Which of the following X-linked conditions is an example of a trinucleotide repeat disorder?

  a. myotonic dystrophy
  b. hemophilia A
  c. hemophilia B
  d. Hunter syndrome

39–33. What percentage of females with full mutations for fragile X syndrome will have some form of mental retardation?

    a. 5
    b. 25
    c. 50
    d. 100

39–34. Which of the following characteristics is NOT a usual manifestation of the fragile X syndrome in affected males?

    a. autism
    b. macro-orchidism
    c. mental retardation
    d. short stature

39–35. Which of the following trinucleotide repeats is associated with the fragile X gene (FMR-1)?

    a. CGG
    b. CAG
    c. GCT
    d. GGG

39–36. What is the best method for detection of both the size of the trinucleotide expansion and methylation of the fragile X gene?

    a. FISH
    b. cytogenetic techniques
    c. PCR
    d. Southern blot

39–37. The gene containing the unstable trinucleotide repeat (ACG) and responsible for myotonic dystrophy is located on what chromosome?

    a. X chromosome
    b. Y chromosome
    c. chromosome 9
    d. chromosome 21

39–38. Which of the following conditions is NOT transmitted via multifactorial inheritance?

    a. ocular albinism
    b. pyloric stenosis
    c. clubfoot
    d. neural tube defect

39–39. Which of the following conditions may be prevented by preconceptional folic acid supplementation?

    a. congenital heart defects
    b. cleft lip
    c. fragile X syndrome
    d. neural tube defects

39–40. What is the recommended preconceptional folic acid dose for a woman with an uncomplicated history planning her first pregnancy?

    a. 400 ng
    b. 400 μg
    c. 4 mg
    d. 4 g

39–41. Which of the following conditions is more common in females than in males?

    a. talipes equinovarus
    b. congenital hip dislocation
    c. ventricular septal defects
    d. pyloric stenosis

39–42. Which of the following conditions is more common in males than in females?

    a. talipes equinovarus
    b. congenital hip dislocation
    c. ventricular septal defects
    d. pyloric stenosis

39–43. What is the risk of cleft lip in a second child of unaffected parents?

    a. 4%
    b. 12%
    c. 25%
    d. 50%

39–44. Approximately what percentage of cases of hydrocephaly are associated with other abnormalities?

    a. 5
    b. 20
    c. 50
    d. 80

39–45. What percentage of cases of hydrocephaly are associated with chromosomal abnormalities?

    a. 1
    b. 10
    c. 28
    d. 80

39–46. Approximately what percentage of males with hydrocephaly from aqueductal stenosis will have inherited the condition by X-linked recessive inheritance?

    a. 10
    b. 25
    c. 50
    d. 100

39–47. Which of the following modes of inheritance is felt to account for the vast majority of cases of renal agenesis (Potter sequence)?

    a. autosomal dominant
    b. autosomal recessive
    c. multifactorial
    d. sporadic or unknown

39–48. Which of the following is most commonly found in newborns with omphaloceles compared with gastroschisis?

    a. defect in abdominal wall to the right of the umbilicus
    b. absence of a hernia sac
    c. intestines covered with a thickened inflammatory exudate
    d. high percentage of chromosomal and other abnormalities

39–49. Approximately how many genes are contained in each human nucleus?

    a. 5000 to 10,000
    b. 50,000 to 100,000
    c. 5 million to 10 million
    d. 10 million to 10 billion

39–50. What is the in vitro technique in which large amounts of specific DNA sequences can be synthesized over a relatively short period of time?

    a. Southern blotting
    b. restriction endonuclease reaction
    c. polymerase chain reactions
    d. allele-specific oligonucleotide reaction

Prenatal Diagnosis and Invasive Techniques to Monitor the Fetus

40–1. A woman who ingests excessive amounts of which of the following vitamins would benefit from preconceptional counseling?

    a. folic acid
    b. vitamin C
    c. vitamin A
    d. vitamin B_6

40–2. Evaluation of malformed infants who die in the perinatal period should include all but which of the following?

    a. autopsy
    b. radiographic skeletal survey
    c. chromosomal analysis
    d. amount of tobacco and caffeine exposure

40–3. Which of the following structures is NOT involved in the synthesis of alpha-fetoprotein (AFP), a glycoprotein synthesized by the fetus?

   a. bone marrow
   b. yolk sac
   c. gastrointestinal tract
   d. liver

40–4. AFP concentration is highest in both fetal serum and amniotic fluid at what week of gestation?

   a. 7th
   b. 11th
   c. 13th
   d. 17th

40–5. Which of the following conditions is associated with an elevated level of maternal serum AFP?

   a. gestational trophoblastic disease
   b. increased maternal weight
   c. overestimated gestational age
   d. cystic hygroma

40–6. Which of the following is most likely associated with a low maternal serum AFP level?

   a. sacrococcygeal teratoma
   b. polycystic kidney
   c. omphalocele
   d. chromosomal trisomies

40–7. Concentrations of AFP are measured in nanograms (ng) in which of the following?

   a. fetal serum
   b. fetal urine
   c. amnionic fluid
   d. maternal serum

40–8. Amnionic fluid acetylcholinesterase levels are most useful in the detection of which condition?

   a. chromosomal trisomies
   b. fetal death
   c. overestimation of gestational age
   d. fetal blood contamination

40–9. What is the risk of an affected offspring if one parent has a neural tube defect?

   a. 2-fold increase
   b. 4-fold increase

   c. 10-fold increase
   d. 20-fold increase

40–10. What percentage of neural tube defects occur in women with no risk factors?

   a. 1
   b. 20
   c. 50
   d. 90

40–11. What is the recommended dose of folic acid supplementation preconceptionally in a woman who has a previous child with a neural tube defect?

   a. 0.4 ng
   b. 0.4 µg
   c. 0.4 mg
   d. 4.0 mg

40–12. What is the approximate decrease in neural tube defects with folic acid supplementation?

   a. 10%
   b. 25%
   c. 70%
   d. 99%

40–13. The likelihood of a neural tube defect associated with an elevated maternal serum AFP is decreased by approximately what percentage if the ultrasound screening is normal?

   a. 50
   b. 70
   c. 90
   d. 100

40–14. What percentage of fetuses with spina bifida will have some type of cranial anomaly detected by ultrasound (i.e., "lemon sign," ventriculomegaly, etc.)?

   a. 99
   b. 58
   c. 25
   d. 5

40–15. What percentage of fetuses with isolated neural tube defects will have aneuploidy?

   a. 1 to 2
   b. 5 to 6
   c. 25 to 30
   d. 55 to 60

40–16. Which of the following is NOT associated with an unexplained elevated maternal serum AFP at 16 weeks' gestation?

    a. closed neural tube defect
    b. perinatal mortality
    c. placental abruption
    d. fetal death

40–17. What percentage of Down syndrome fetuses are born to women under the age of 35 years?

    a. 10
    b. 30
    c. 60
    d. 80

40–18. What percentage of all Down syndrome fetuses can be diagnosed prenatally by providing amniocentesis to all women age 35 years or older and to those younger than 35 whose age-adjusted AFP level indicates a risk of 1 in 270 or greater?

    a. 5 to 10
    b. 20 to 30
    c. 45 to 50
    d. 75 to 80

40–19. Which of the following markers is not included in the "triple screen" for Down syndrome?

    a. maternal serum AFP
    b. placental lactogen
    c. unconjugated estriol
    d. chorionic gonadotropin

40–20. What percentage of fetuses with Down syndrome can be detected utilizing the "triple screen"?

    a. 25
    b. 60 to 70
    c. 80 to 90
    d. 100

40–21. Which of the following aneuploidies is associated with a decrease in all three serum markers?

    a. trisomy 18
    b. trisomy 13
    c. trisomy 21
    d. monosomy X

40–22. What proportion of African-Americans are heterozygous for the sickle cell gene?

    a. 1 in 4
    b. 1 in 12
    c. 1 in 24
    d. 1 in 42

40–23. What proportion of Ashkenazi Jews are heterozygous for Tay-Sachs disease?

    a. 1 in 10
    b. 1 in 30
    c. 1 in 75
    d. 1 in 150

40–24. The gene mutation DF508 on chromosome 7 is responsible for which of the following conditions?

    a. cystic fibrosis
    b. Tay–Sachs disease
    c. sickle cell disease
    d. Hunter disease

40–25. Deficiency of the enzyme, hexosaminidase A, is associated with which condition?

    a. cystic fibrosis
    b. Tay–Sachs disease
    c. sickle cell disease
    d. Hunter disease

40–26. What percentage of Caucasians are carriers for cystic fibrosis?

    a. 1
    b. 4
    c. 8
    d. 12

40–27. Which of the following dyes is recommended to distinguish separate sacs when performing amniocentesis in twin gestations?

    a. indigo carmine
    b. nile blue
    c. cardiac green
    d. methylene blue

40–28. Which of the following dyes has been reported to cause hemolytic anemia and methemoglobinemia when utilized for amniocentesis?

    a. indigo carmine
    b. nile blue
    c. cardiac green
    d. methylene blue

40–29. What is the percentage of success in obtaining amnionic fluid with early amniocentesis (i.e., prior to 15 weeks' gestation)?

    a. 50
    b. 65
    c. 85
    d. >95

40–30. What is the increase in pregnancy loss with CVS and early amniocentesis compared with midtrimester amniocentesis?

    a. 2.5-fold
    b. 3- to 4-fold
    c. 6.5-fold
    d. 10-fold

40–31. Which is the major technical problem with chorionic villus sampling compared to amniocentesis?

    a. failure to obtain sample
    b. failure of sample to grow

    c. increased chromosomal mosaicism
    d. overgrowth of maternal cells

40–32. Which of the following has been reported to be associated with an increase in severe limb abnormalities?

    a. chorionic villus sampling performed at 8 to 9 weeks
    b. chorionic villus sampling performed at 9 to 12 weeks
    c. amniocentesis performed at 9 to 12 weeks
    d. amniocentesis performed at 13 to 15 weeks

40–33. When performing percutaneous umbilical blood sampling (cordocentesis), where is the umbilical cord usually punctured?

    a. 1 to 2 cm from placental insertion
    b. 1 to 2 cm from fetal insertion
    c. 3 to 4 cm from placental insertion
    d. 3 to 4 cm from fetal insertion

40–34. The early fetal loss from cordocentesis has been reported to be approximately what percentage?

    a. <0.5
    b. 1
    c. 3
    d. 5

41

Drugs and Medications

41–1. Which of the following represents the ovum period?

    a. prefertilization
    b. fertilization to implantation
    c. fertilization through the 4th week
    d. fertilization through the 8th week

41–2. Which of the following represents the embryonic period?

    a. fertilization through 6 weeks
    b. implantation through 8 weeks
    c. 2nd through 8th week
    d. 1st through 12th week

41–3. Which of the following represents the fetal period?

    a. implantation through 8 weeks
    b. implantation through 12 weeks
    c. 8 weeks until term
    d. 12 weeks until term

41–4. Which of the following periods is most critical with regard to malformations?

    a. prefertilization
    b. zygote (ovum)
    c. embryonic
    d. fetal

41–5. Tetracycline is most likely to cause a significant problem when taken during which of the following periods?

    a. prefertilization
    b. ovum
    c. embryonic
    d. fetal

41–6. Which of the following drugs is NOT a known or suspected teratogen?

    a. isotretinoin
    b. etretinate
    c. diethylstilbestrol
    d. metronidazole

41–7. There are approximately how many documented human teratogens?

    a. 5
    b. 30
    c. 500
    d. 1500

41–8. Which of the following drugs is best known as a litogen?

    a. Bendectin®
    b. lithium
    c. heparin
    d. tetracycline

41–9. What is the FDA category for drugs for which controlled studies in humans have demonstrated no fetal risk?

    a. A
    b. B
    c. C
    d. D

41–10. What is the FDA category for drugs for which there are no adequate studies available?

    a. B
    b. C
    c. D
    d. X

41–11. Which of the following drugs is an FDA category X drug?

    a. coumarin
    b. isotretinoin
    c. acyclovir
    d. diazepam

41–12. What is the correlation between the FDA classification of drugs (i.e., A,B,C,D, and X) and actual teratogenic risk?

    a. excellent
    b. good
    c. fair
    d. poor

41–13. Which of the following antibiotics has poor access to the fetus when given to the mother?

    a. penicillin
    b. erythromycin
    c. cephalosporins
    d. tetracyclines

41–14. Which of the following antibiotics given to the mother near delivery may result in significant hyperbilirubinemia in the newborn?

    a. penicillin
    b. cephalosporin
    c. clindamycin
    d. sulfonamides

41–15. Which of the following antibiotics is an alternative to an aminoglycoside?

    a. aztreonam
    b. clindamycin
    c. sulfonamide
    d. clindamycin

41–16. Which of the following antibiotics is a folate antagonist?

    a. trimethoprim
    b. nitrofurantoin
    c. tetracycline
    d. erythromycin

41–17. Which of the following antibiotics is the drug of choice for *Clostridium dificile* pseudomembranous colitis?

    a. ampicillin
    b. vancomycin
    c. aztreonam
    d. imipenem

41–18. Which of the following antibiotics has been reported to cause irreversible arthropathy in immature animals?

    a. fluoroquinolones
    b. vancomycin
    c. nitrofurantoin
    d. sulfonamides

41–19. Which of the following antibiotics is useful for the treatment of *Mycobacterium avium* complex (MAC) in patients with HIV infection?

    a. streptomycin
    b. vancomycin
    c. isoniazid
    d. rifabutin

41–20. Which of the following antifungal agents has been reported to possibly be associated with conjoined twins in humans and skeletal and central nervous system defects in animal studies?

    a. nystatin
    b. clotrimazole
    c. amphotericin B
    d. griseofulvin

41–21. Which of the following drugs has been utilized to prevent fetal HIV transmission?

    a. ddC
    b. d4T
    c. AZT
    d. 3TC

41–22. Which of the following antiviral drugs is utilized to prevent or modify influenza infections?

    a. acyclovir
    b. ganciclovir
    c. ribavirin
    d. amantadine

41–23. Which of the following antiviral agents is NOT recommended for use in pregnant women because it has been shown to produce hydrocephalus and limb anomalies in animal models?

    a. zidovudine (AZT)
    b. acyclovir
    c. amantidine
    d. ribavirin

41–24. Although not generally recommended for use in early pregnancy because of the potential for being mutagenic and carcinogenic, which of the following antiparasitic agents has been shown to produce no adverse effects in over 1000 infants who were exposed to it in the first trimester?

    a. metronidazole
    b. lindane
    c. pyrimethamine
    d. spiramycin

41–25. Which of the following antibiotics has been utilized for the treatment of toxoplasmosis?

    a. lindane
    b. chloroquine
    c. spiramycin
    d. metronidazole

41–26. Which of the following antihypertensives may cause accumulation of cyanide in the fetal liver?

    a. methyldopa
    b. nitroprusside
    c. labetolol
    d. nifedipine

41–27. Which of the following antihypertensives has been reported to be associated with congenital hypocalvaria, renal anomalies, nephrotoxicity, and neonatal anuria?

    a. sodium nitroprusside
    b. captopril
    c. clonidine
    d. labetolol

41–28. Which of the following diuretics has the theoretical potential for causing feminization of male fetuses?

    a. spironolactone
    b. ethacrynic acid
    c. acetazolamide
    d. hydrochlorothiazide

41–29. What is the approximate molecular weight of enoxapanin (low-molecular-weight heparin)?

    a. 365
    b. 1000
    c. 4000
    d. 20,000

41–30. Which of the following abnormalities is NOT part of the fetal warfarin syndrome?

    a. nasal hypoplasia
    b. stippled bone epiphyses
    c. anencephaly
    d. microcephaly

41–31. Which of the following anticonvulsant medications is NOT associated with the "anticonvulsant embryopathy"?

    a. phenytoin
    b. carbamazepine
    c. trimethadione
    d. phenobarbital

41–32. What is the estimated risk of spina bifida from first-trimester valproic acid exposure?

    a. 1 to 2%
    b. 5 to 10%
    c. 20 to 25%
    d. 30 to 40%

41–33. Which of the following psychotropic drugs has been reported to be associated with an increased risk of fetal cardiovascular anomalies, especially Ebstein anomaly?

    a. amitriptyline
    b. imipramine
    c. lithium
    d. chlorpromazine

41–34. Which of the following antidepressants belongs to the selective serotonin reuptake inhibitor (SSRI) class?

    a. lithium
    b. nortriptyline
    c. monamine oxidase inhibitors
    d. fluoxetine

41–35. Which of the following analgesics has been reported to be associated with constriction of the fetus ductus arteriosus?

    a. aspirin
    b. indomethacin
    c. acetaminophen
    d. butorphanol

41–36. Which of the following antineoplastic agents has been reported to be associated with the highest rate of malformations?

    a. cyclophosphamide
    b. busulfan
    c. aminopterin
    d. methotrexate

41–37. Which of the following vitamins has been reported to cause congenital malformations if given in excess amounts?

    a. vitamin D
    b. vitamin K
    c. vitamin A
    d. vitamin B_{12}

41–38. Which of the following has not been reported to be associated with an increase in congenital malformations?

    a. isotretinoin
    b. vitamin A
    c. etretinate
    d. tretinoin

41–39. Which of the following compounds is both teratogenic and has been detected in serum up to 2 years after cessation of therapy?

   a. isotretinoin
   b. etretinate
   c. tretinoin
   d. vitamin A

41–40. Which of the following hormones may cause virilization of the female fetus?

   a. clomid
   b. danazol

   c. prednisone
   d. provera

41–41. Which of the following social or illicit substances is associated with the syndrome manifested by mental retardation, cardiac defects, spinal defects, and craniofacial anomalies?

   a. alcohol
   b. amphetamines
   c. lysergic acid
   d. heroin

42

Diseases and Injuries of the Fetus and Newborn

42–1. Which of the following is NOT a sign of hyaline membrane disease (RDS)?

   a. increased respiratory rate
   b. chest wall retraction during inspiration
   c. grunting
   d. hypertension

42–2. A diffuse reticulogranular infiltrate and an air bronchogram on chest x-ray is most common in which disorder of the newborn?

   a. idiopathic respiratory distress syndrome
   b. pneumonia
   c. meconium aspiration
   d. heart failure

42–3. Surfactant therapy is most efficacious for prevention or reduction of which of the following?

   a. persistent ductus arteriosus
   b. bronchopulmonary dysplasia

   c. intraventricular hemorrhage
   d. neonatal oxygen requirements

42–4. Which of the following is a complication of surfactant therapy?

   a. pulmonary hemorrhage
   b. intraventricular hemorrhage
   c. pneumonitis
   d. persistent ductus arteriosus

42–5. Which of the following is a complication of hyperoxia?

   a. pulmonary hemorrhage
   b. retinopathy
   c. pneumonitis
   d. intraventricular hemorrhage

42–6. At approximately what week does the concentration of lecithin relative to sphingomyelin begin to rise?

   a. 28th
   b. 32nd

c. 34th
d. 36th

42–7. Which of the following tests is least likely to be affected by contaminants such as blood, meconium, or vaginal secretions?

a. lecithin–sphingomyelin ratio
b. phosphatidylglycerol measurement
c. foam stability test
d. fluorescent polarization

42–8. A positive "shake test" (foam stability test) is usually correlated with what level of L/S ratio?

a. 1.5
b. 2.0
c. 4.0
d. 12.0

42–9. Which of the following tests is used to measure the surfactant–albumin ratio in uncentrifuged amnionic fluid?

a. fluorescent polarization
b. amnionic fluid absorbance at 650 nm
c. DPPC
d. TDx-FLM

42–10. Which of the following vitamins has been utilized in an attempt to prevent retrolental fibroplasia (retinopathy of prematurity)?

a. vitamin A
b. vitamin K
c. vitamin E
d. vitamin D

42–11. Approximately what percentage of pregnancies are complicated by meconium-stained fluid?

a. 1
b. 10
c. 20
d. 30

42–12. Which of the following mechanisms is felt to be responsible for the pathophysiologic manifestations seen with meconium aspiration syndrome?

a. mechanical blockage by meconium
b. direct chemical damage by meconium
c. meconium pneumonitis
d. chronic fetal asphyxia

42–13. Which of the following markers is most likely to be abnormal in the umbilical cord blood of newborns with meconium-stained fluid?

a. pH
b. erythropoietin
c. hypoxanthine
d. lactate

42–14. Which of the following heart-rate patterns is most likely to predict meconium aspiration?

a. variable decelerations
b. saltatory
c. late decelerations
d. none of the above

42–15. Most intraventricular hemorrhages of the preterm infant develop by which of the following time periods?

a. first hour of birth
b. first 24 hours after birth
c. first 72 hours after birth
d. first 7 days after birth

42–16. Which of the following factors best correlates with the presence of intraventricular hemorrhage?

a. prematurity
b. length of labor
c. forceps delivery
d. late decelerations

42–17. Approximately what percentage of all neonates born before 34 weeks will have evidence of intraventricular hemorrhage?

a. 2
b. 10
c. 20
d. 50

42–18. Approximately what percentage of asymptomatic term neonates have sonographic evidence of subependymal hemorrhage?

a. <1
b. 4
c. 18
d. 33

42–19. Which grade of intraventricular hemorrhage is associated with ventricular dilation?

   a. I
   b. II
   c. III
   d. IV

42–20. Which of the following has NOT been associated with intraventricular hemorrhage?

   a. respiratory distress syndrome
   b. mechanical ventilation
   c. hypoxia
   d. labor

42–21. Which of the following has been proven to reduce the risk of intraventricular hemorrhage?

   a. vitamin K
   b. vitamin E
   c. phenobarbital
   d. corticosteroids

42–22. Which is the most common form of cerebral palsy?

   a. diplegic type
   b. hemiplegic type
   c. quadriplegic type
   d. extrapyramidal type

42–23. What percentage of cerebral palsy cases are associated with mental retardation?

   a. 1
   b. 10
   c. 25
   d. 60

42–24. What is the approximate incidence of cerebral palsy in the United States?

   a. 1 to 2 per 100 live births
   b. 1 to 2 per 1000 live births
   c. 1 to 2 per 10,000 live births
   d. 3 to 5 per 10,000 live births

42–25. What is the incidence of cerebral palsy in low-birthweight (<2500 g) infants?

   a. 15 per 100 live births
   b. 15 per 1000 live births
   c. 15 per 10,000 live births
   d. 15 per 100,000 live births

42–26. What has happened to the incidence of cerebral palsy over the last two decades?

   a. slightly decreased
   b. markedly decreased
   c. markedly increased
   d. essentially unchanged

42–27. Which of the following factors is NOT strongly predictive of the presence of cerebral palsy in the newborn?

   a. forceps delivery
   b. maternal mental retardation
   c. birthweight less than 2000 g
   d. fetal malformations

42–28. What percentage of cerebral palsy can be attributed to asphyxia?

   a. 10
   b. 30
   c. 50
   d. 75

42–29. Which of the following is the best predictor of cerebral palsy?

   a. Apgar score
   b. abnormal fetal heart rate pattern
   c. neonatal acidosis
   d. neonatal encephalopathy

42–30. What percentage of low-birthweight newborns with cerebral palsy had a grade III or IV intraventricular hemorrhage at birth?

   a. 5
   b. 28
   c. 40
   d. 94

42–31. What is the increased risk of cerebral palsy in low-birthweight newborns with grade III or IV intraventricular hemorrhage compared with controls or those with only a grade I or II hemorrhage?

   a. 2-fold
   b. 8-fold
   c. 16-fold
   d. 100-fold

42–32. In a recent review of over 200 neurologically impaired neonates, what percentage were classified as nonpreventable?

  a. 10
  b. 25
  c. 50
  d. 75

42–33. What is the umbilical artery pH cutoff that best defines significant newborn acidemia?

  a. 7.20
  b. 7.15
  c. 7.10
  d. 7.00

42–34. What percentage of newborns with mild encephalopathy can be expected to have abnormal neurological development?

  a. 0
  b. 20
  c. 50
  d. 80

42–35. What percentage of newborns with moderate encephalopathy can be expected to develop normally neurologically?

  a. 0
  b. 20
  c. 50
  d. 80

42–36. What are the most common causes of cerebral palsy?

  a. prenatal factors
  b. perinatal factors
  c. postnatal factors
  d. unknown

42–37. What is the incidence of severe mental retardation?

  a. 3 per 100
  b. 3 per 1000
  c. 3 per 10,000
  d. 3 per 100,000

42–38. What is the approximate mean cord hemoglobin concentration at term?

  a. 10 g/dL
  b. 13 g/dL

  c. 17 g/dL
  d. 21 g/dL

42–39. Of the following, which is the most likely cause of fetal-to-maternal hemorrhage?

  a. chorioangioma
  b. placental abruption
  c. placenta previa
  d. oxytocin-induced labor

42–40. What is the chance that a D-negative woman delivered of a D-positive but ABO-compatible infant will be D-isoimmunized postpartum?

  a. 1%
  b. 5%
  c. 16%
  d. 33%

42–41. What is the chance that a D-negative woman delivered of a D-positive but ABO-incompatible infant will be D-isoimmunized by 6 months postpartum?

  a. 2%
  b. 12%
  c. 20%
  d. 42%

42–42. The CDE antigens are inherited independent of other blood group antigens and are located on which chromosome?

  a. 1
  b. 21
  c. X
  d. Y

42–43. Which of the following ethnic groups have the highest incidence of D-negativity?

  a. African-Americans
  b. white Americans
  c. American Indians
  d. Basques

42–44. What percentage of newborns have ABO maternal blood group incompatibility?

  a. 1
  b. 10
  c. 20
  d. 50

42–45. Which of the following red cell antigens does NOT cause hemolytic disease of the newborn?

    a. CDE
    b. Kell
    c. Duffy
    d. Lewis

42–46. Which of the following is NOT one of the criteria for confirming the diagnosis of ABO incompatibility?

    a. mother is blood group O
    b. fetus is blood group A or B
    c. onset of jaundice after 7 days
    d. varying degrees of anemia, reticulocytosis, and erythroblastosis

42–47. What percentage of pregnant women will have atypical red cell antibodies?

    a. 1
    b. 5
    c. 15
    d. 20

42–48. What is the most common atypical red cell antibody encountered?

    a. anti-Lewis
    b. anti-Kell
    c. anti-Duffy
    d. anti-Kidd

42–49. How is detection of maternal antibodies that have been absorbed by fetal cells best accomplished?

    a. indirect Coombs test
    b. direct Coombs test
    c. rosette test
    d. enzyme-linked antiglobulin test

42–50. The severity of ascites seen with hydrops fetalis is best correlated with which of the following?

    a. portal hypertension
    b. degree and severity of anemia
    c. hypoproteinemia
    d. decreased colloid oncotic pressure

42–51. Which of the following fetal heart rate patterns is characteristic of fetuses with severe anemia?

    a. late decelerations
    b. variable decelerations
    c. sinusoidal pattern
    d. absence of variability

42–52. Approximately what percentage of D-negative women having early elective abortions become isoimmunized without D-immunoglobulin?

    a. <1
    b. 5
    c. 25
    d. 33

42–53. One dose of 300 mg of D-immunoglobulin will protect the mother against a bleed of approximately how much fetal blood?

    a. 5 mL
    b. 30 mL
    c. 90 mL
    d. 150 mL

42–54. What would be the expected hemoglobin in a fetus whose delta OD values from amniocentesis are in upper zone 2?

    a. 16 g/dL
    b. 14 to 16 g/dL
    c. 11.0 to 13.9 g/dL
    d. 8.0 to 10.9 g/dL

42–55. With D-isoimmunization, when the hemoglobin deficit obtained by fetal cord blood sampling exceeds 2 g/dL from the mean for normal fetuses of corresponding gestational age, what is the recommended next step?

    a. repeat sample in 1 week
    b. repeat sample in 2 weeks
    c. perform amniocentesis for optical density determination
    d. begin fetal transfusions

42–56. What is the approximate survival rate for fetuses who undergo intravascular transfusions for D-isoimmunization?

    a. 20%
    b. 33%

c. 65%
d. 85%

42–57. What type blood is utilized for initial exchange transfusion in the anemic newborn?

 a. O, D-negative
 b. O, D-positive
 c. maternal blood type, D-positive
 d. AB, D-negative

42–58. In the otherwise uncomplicated newborn, what is the unconjugated bilirubin level above which kernicterus is likely to develop?

 a. 3 mg/dL
 b. 7 mg/dL
 c. 15 to 16 mg/dL
 d. 18 to 20 mg/dL

42–59. Which of the following compounds excreted into breast milk has been associated with jaundice of the newborn?

 a. 17α-hydroxylase
 b. pregnane 3α, 20, β-diol
 c. pregnenolone
 d. androstenedione

42–60. With physiological jaundice, what is the maximum level that serum bilirubin reaches?

 a. 2 mg/dL
 b. 5 mg/dL
 c. 10 mg/dL
 d. 18 mg/dL

42–61. Which of the following has NOT been utilized to lower the newborn serum level of bilirubin?

 a. phenobarbital
 b. fluorescent light
 c. vitamin K
 d. exchange transfusion

42–62. What percentage of fetuses with nonimmune hydrops are idiopathic?

 a. ~10
 b. ~20
 c. ~50
 d. ~70

42–63. Which of the following intrinsic lesions is most commonly associated with nonimmune hydrops?

 a. cystic hygroma
 b. cardiac anomalies
 c. sacrococcygeal teratoma
 d. twin–twin transfusion

42–64. Which of the following fetal cardiac arrhythmias is most likely to be associated with nonimmune hydrops?

 a. supraventricular tachycardia (>200 bpm)
 b. bradycardia (<110 bpm)
 c. second-degree heart block
 d. ventricular extrasystole

42–65. What is the most likely cause of hemorrhagic disease of the newborn?

 a. autosomal dominant
 b. autosomal recessive
 c. maternal anticoagulation
 d. neonatal deficiency of vitamin K

42–66. What is the most likely diagnosis when the newborn has severe thrombocytopenia but the mother has a normal platelet count?

 a. immunological thrombocytopenia
 b. preeclampsia–eclampsia
 c. isoimmune thrombocytopenia
 d. maternal drug ingestion

42–67. Which of the following is NOT a common clinical finding in newborns with necrotizing enterocolitis?

 a. pneumatosis intestinalis
 b. abdominal distention
 c. meconium stools
 d. ileus

42–68. What is the most common type of intracranial hemorrhage encountered in the preterm newborn?

 a. intraventricular
 b. cortical
 c. periventricular
 d. subdural

42–69. What is the most common cause of intracranial hemorrhage?

    a. preterm birth
    b. birth trauma
    c. infection
    d. medication

42–70. Which is the focal swelling of the scalp from edema fluid overlying the periosteum?

    a. cephalohematoma
    b. caput succedaneum
    c. periosteal hematoma
    d. caput periosteum

42–71. What is the approximate incidence in term births of brachial plexus injury?

    a. 1 in 12
    b. 1 in 100
    c. 1 in 500
    d. 1 in 3000

42–72. What percentage of brachial plexus injuries occur in macrosomic infants?

    a. 5
    b. 30

    c. 60
    d. 75

42–73. Approximately what percentage of facial paralysis injuries occur with spontaneous delivery?

    a. 1
    b. 11
    c. 22
    d. 33

42–74. What is the approximate incidence of clavicular fracture in live births?

    a. 0.3%
    b. 0.1 to 0.2%
    c. 1.0 to 2.0%
    d. 3.5%

42–75. Torticollis is more commonly associated with which of the following delivery modes?

    a. spontaneous vertex
    b. breech extraction
    c. forceps
    d. cesarean section

Techniques Used to Assess Fetal Health

43

Antepartum Assessment

43–1. How early in gestation does passive unstimulated activity (movement) of the human fetus commence?

  a. 3 weeks
  b. 7 weeks
  c. 11 weeks
  d. 15 weeks

43–2. What is the longest time period during which fetal body movements are absent?

  a. 5 min
  b. 13 min
  c. 30 min
  d. 90 min

43–3. Continuous eye movements in the absence of body movements and no accelerations of the fetal heart is consistent with which of the following fetal behavioral states?

  a. 1F
  b. 2F
  c. 3F
  d. 4F

43–4. What is the mean length of the quiet or inactive state for term fetuses (i.e., "sleep cyclicity")?

  a. 11 min
  b. 23 min
  c. 75 min
  d. 105 min

43–5. What percentage of fetal body movements (recorded by Doppler device) will be perceived by the mother after 36 weeks?

  a. 16
  b. 38
  c. 65
  d. 90

43–6. What is the range of normal weekly counts of fetal movement?

  a. 20 to 600
  b. 20 to 950
  c. 50 to 600
  d. 50 to 950

43–7. When obtaining fetal movement records, which is a commonly used definition of abnormal activity?

    a. less than 10 movements/12 hr
    b. less than 20 movements/12 hr
    c. less than 40 movements/12 hr
    d. less than 60 movements/12 hr

43–8. In normal fetuses, what is the length of time that fetal breathing movements may be totally absent?

    a. 20 min
    b. 60 min
    c. 120 min
    d. 200 min

43–9. Irregular bursts of fetal breathing occur at which rate?

    a. 60 cycles/min
    b. 120 cycles/min
    c. 240 cycles/min
    d. 360 cycles/min

43–10. Which of the following variables is associated with absent fetal breathing movements?

    a. maternal meals
    b. decreased fetal heart rate
    c. sound stimuli
    d. labor

43–11. What is the false-positive rate for a contraction stress test?

    a. 1%
    b. 8%
    c. 15%
    d. 25 to 75%

43–12. What is the false-negative rate of a contraction stress test?

    a. 1%
    b. 5%
    c. 15%
    d. 50%

43–13. What controls fetal heart rate acceleration?

    a. autonomic function
    b. aortic baroreceptor reflexes
    c. carotid baroreceptor reflexes
    d. humeral factors such as atrial natriuretic peptide

43–14. At what gestational age should 90 percent or more of fetuses be expected to have fetal heart rate accelerations with movement?

    a. 24 weeks
    b. 28 weeks
    c. 32 weeks
    d. 36 weeks

43–15. What is the ACOG definition of a reactive NST?

    a. 1 acceleration in 20 min
    b. 2 accelerations in 20 min
    c. 5 or more accelerations in 20 min
    d. 6 or more accelerations in 20 min

43–16. When fetal heart rate accelerations are insignificant, false positive nonstress tests approach what level?

    a. 2%
    b. 10%
    c. 20%
    d. 90%

43–17. What is the associated perinatal pathology for the fetus with a nonreactive NST for 90 minutes?

    a. 10%
    b. 25%
    c. 50%
    d. 90%

43–18. What is the minimal level of sound necessary to evoke fetal movements?

    a. 50 dB
    b. 100 dB
    c. 500 dB
    d. 1000 dB

43–19. Which of the following is NOT a biophysical variable commonly used in the biophysical profile test?

    a. fetal heart rate acceleration
    b. fetal breathing
    c. fetal movement
    d. fetal urination

43–20. What is the false-normal rate for the biophysical profile test?

    a. 1 in 10
    b. 1 in 100

c. 1 in 1000
d. 1 in 10,000

43–21. Which of the following best describes a biophysical score of 6?

    a. normal score
    b. equivocal score
    c. abnormal score
    d. acidotic score

43–22. Doppler velocimetry may be useful in which of the following conditions?

    a. growth retardation
    b. diabetes
    c. preeclampsia
    d. lupus

43–23. What is the single best test of fetal well-being?

    a. CST
    b. NST
    c. doppler velocimetry
    d. There is no single best test.

43–24. What is the incidence of cerebral palsy when the biophysical profile is 10?

    a. 0.8 per 1000
    b. 2.0 per 1000
    c. 3.0 per 10,000
    d. 3.0 per 100,000

44

Doppler and Ultrasound

44–1. What is the major biological hazard from fetal ultrasound?

    a. none
    b. early spontaneous abortions
    c. impaired neonatal hearing
    d. chromosomal breakage

44–2. What do the transducers employed in real-time ultrasonography generate?

    a. single-pulse echo systems
    b. multiple-pulse echo systems activated at random
    c. multiple-pulse echo systems activated in sequence
    d. dual-pulse echo systems activated at random

44–3. What energy level for ultrasound has the FDA limited during fetal exposure?

    a. 10 mW per cm^2
    b. 55 mW per cm^2
    c. 94 mW per cm^2
    d. 200 mW per cm^2

44–4. In the RADIUS trial, what was the major conclusion regarding routine ultrasound?

    a. Adverse perinatal outcomes were reduced.
    b. Preterm delivery was reduced.
    c. Fetal growth restriction was reduced.
    d. Perinatal outcome was not improved.

44–5. What is the preferred fetal dimension for estimating gestational age at 8 to 10 weeks of pregnancy?

    a. femur length
    b. crown–rump length
    c. biparietal diameter
    d. humerus length

44–6. Using transabdominal sonography, when is the gestational sac reliably seen (menstrual age)?

    a. 4 weeks
    b. 6 weeks
    c. 8 weeks
    d. 9 weeks

44–7. Using transvaginal screening, when is the gestational sac (menstrual age) usually seen?

    a. 3 weeks
    b. 5 weeks
    c. 7 weeks
    d. 8 weeks

44–8. What is the overall sensitivity of sonography in detecting fetal defects?

    a. 29%
    b. 53%
    c. 76%
    d. 99%

44–9. Which of the following sonographic views is used to measure the biparietal diameter and head circumference?

    a. transthalamic
    b. transventricular
    c. transcerebellar
    d. transhemispheric

44–10. What is the incidence of hydrocephalus?

    a. 0.3 to 0.8 per 100 births
    b. 0.3 to 0.8 per 1000 births
    c. 0.3 to 0.8 per 10,000 births
    d. 0.3 to 0.8 per 100,000 births

44–11. What is the average diameter of the lateral ventricular atrium between 15 and 35 weeks?

    a. 2 to 3 mm
    b. 5 to 7 mm
    c. 6 to 9 mm
    d. 12 to 15 mm

44–12. A free-floating or dangling choroid plexus is suggestive of which of the following diagnoses?

    a. hydrocephalus
    b. aqueductal stenosis
    c. choroid plexus cyst
    d. cerebral atrophy

44–13. What is the accuracy of diagnosing anencephaly in the second trimester?

    a. 25%
    b. 50%
    c. 75%
    d. 100%

44–14. The presence of an encephalocele is an important feature of which of the following syndromes?

    a. Meckel–Gruber
    b. Hunter
    c. Hurler
    d. Edward

44–15. Which of the following signs describes frontal bone scalloping?

    a. lemon sign
    b. apple sign
    c. pear sign
    d. banana sign

44–16. Cerebral ventriculomegaly occurs in approximately what percentage of fetuses with spina bifida?

    a. 10
    b. 50
    c. 80
    d. 100

44–17. What percentage of second-trimester fetuses will have a choroid plexus cyst?

    a. 3
    b. 7
    c. 14
    d. 19

44–18. What is the most common chromosomal abnormality associated with a choroid plexus cyst?

    a. trisomy 21
    b. trisomy 13
    c. trisomy 18
    d. triploidy

44–19. What is the most common chromosomal anomaly associated with cystic hygromas in second- or third-trimester fetuses?

    a. trisomy 21
    b. trisomy 18

c. monosomy X

d. triploidy

44–20. What is the incidence of congenital heart disease?

    a. 8 per 100

    b. 8 per 1000

    c. 8 per 10,000

    d. 8 per 30,000

44–21. What percentage of fetuses with congenital heart defects is associated with aneuploidy?

    a. 1

    b. 9

    c. 17

    d. 32

44–22. What is the positive predictive value of ultrasound for the detection of congenital heart defects?

    a. 25%

    b. 55%

    c. 75%

    d. 99%

44–23. What is the most specific finding in fetuses with diaphragmatic hernias?

    a. cystic structure behind the left atrium

    b. absence of intra-abdominal stomach bubble

    c. small abdominal circumference

    d. peristalsis in the fetal chest

44–24. What percentage of fetuses with a diaphragmatic hernia will have other associated major anomalies?

    a. 1

    b. 10

    c. 50

    d. 75

44–25. In what percentage of fetuses is it possible to visualize the fetal stomach after 14 weeks?

    a. 5

    b. 25

    c. 76

    d. 98

44–26. What percentage of fetuses with esophageal atresia or tracheoesophageal fistula will have associated anomalies?

    a. 5

    b. 25

    c. 50

    d. 78

44–27. What percentage of fetuses with the "double-bubble sign" (duodenal atresia) will have trisomy 21?

    a. 5

    b. 18

    c. 30

    d. 55

44–28. The fetal kidneys can routinely be visualized by what gestational age?

    a. 8 weeks

    b. 12 weeks

    c. 18 weeks

    d. 22 weeks

44–29. What is the average urine output (per hr) in a fetus at term?

    a. 5 mL

    b. 20 mL

    c. 33 mL

    d. 50 mL

44–30. Which of the following characteristics is NOT associated with Potter syndrome?

    a. pulmonary hypoplasia

    b. limb deformities

    c. tight skin

    d. abnormal fascies

44–31. How is the infantile polycystic kidney disease inherited?

    a. autosomal dominant

    b. autosomal recessive

    c. multifactorial

    d. sporadic

44–32. What is the uterine blood flow at term?

    a. 50 mL per min

    b. 100 to 150 mL per min

    c. 300 to 425 mL per min

    d. 500 to 750 mL per min

44–33. Doppler velocimetry has proven to be of benefit in which of the following conditions?

    a. fetal growth restriction
    b. fetal hypoxia
    c. fetal distress
    d. pregnancy-induced hypertension

44–34. In which of the following arteries is the systolic–diastolic (S/D) ratio measured?

    a. fetal umbilical artery
    b. fetal carotid artery
    c. fetal aorta
    d. fetal vena cava

44–35. What is the Pourcelot index?

    a. pulsatility index
    b. resistance index
    c. S/D index
    d. reflectance index

44–36. What is the mean fetal cardiac output (per kg per min)?

    a. 50 mL
    b. 100 mL
    c. 230 mL
    d. 425 mL

Section

XIII

Medical and Surgical Complications in Pregnancy

45

General Considerations and Maternal Evaluation

45–1. At which time during pregnancy are most nonobstetrical surgical procedures performed?

   a. 1st trimester
   b. 2nd trimester
   c. 3rd trimester
   d. postpartum

45–2. What are the effects of laparoscopy on the human fetus?

   a. increased congenital anomalies
   b. increased spontaneous abortions
   c. fetal growth restriction
   d. currently unknown

45–3. What type of anesthesia is most commonly employed for nonobstetric surgeries during pregnancy?

   a. epidural
   b. local infiltration
   c. general
   d. regional nerve blocks

45–4. Which of the following neonatal outcomes are affected by surgery (nonobstetrical)?

   a. stillborns
   b. birthweight < 1500 g
   c. congenital malformations
   d. sepsis

45–5. What is the relative risk of leukemia developing in children exposed to x-ray pelvimetry?

  a. 1.0
  b. 1.5
  c. 2.0
  d. 4.0

45–6. Which of the following is an example of radiation of short wavelength and high energy?

  a. x-ray
  b. microwaves
  c. ultrasound
  d. diathermy

45–7. During what period of development is ionizing radiation most likely to cause a lethal effect?

  a. preimplantation
  b. 1st trimester
  c. 2nd trimester
  d. 3rd trimester

45–8. What is the most common type of anomaly seen in humans as a result of exposure to ionizing radiation?

  a. central nervous system
  b. cardiac
  c. limb
  d. renal

45–9. What is the highest estimated risk of mental retardation when the embryo is exposed to radiation of 10 rads at 8 to 15 weeks' gestational age?

  a. 1 to 2%
  b. 4%
  c. 12%
  d. 20%

45–10. What is the risk of congenital malformations, growth retardation, or abortion from exposure to 1 to 5 rads of ionizing radiation at 8 to 15 weeks' gestation?

  a. 1 to 2%
  b. 5%
  c. 8%
  d. not increased

45–11. Approximately how many exposed normal fetuses would have to be aborted to prevent one case of leukemia from a fetal radiation exposure of 1 to 2 rads?

  a. 99
  b. 999
  c. 1999
  d. 19,999

45–12. What is the approximate fetal exposure from a maternal chest x-ray?

  a. <0.1 mrad
  b. 10 mrad
  c. 100 mrad
  d. 1 rad

45–13. What is the average fetal exposure from a single abdominal x-ray film?

  a. <0.1 mrad
  b. 10 mrad
  c. 100 mrad
  d. 1 rad

45–14. A single x-ray film for which of the following delivers the highest dose of radiation to the fetus?

  a. chest
  b. abdomen
  c. rib
  d. hip

45–15. At term, to what dose of radiation is a fetus exposed during a CT scan of the abdomen?

  a. <0.05 rads
  b. 0.1 to 1.0 rad
  c. 1.5 to 2.0 rads
  d. 3.0 to 4.0 rads

45–16. What is the fetal risk from sodium iodine[123]?

  a. minimal perinatal morbidity
  b. moderate perinatal morbidity
  c. severe perinatal morbidity
  d. lethal perinatal morbidity

45–17. What limit has the FDA set for ultrasound energy exposure during fetal imaging?

a. 47 mW/cm^2
b. 94 mW/cm^2
c. 198 mW/cm^2
d. 396 mW/cm^2

45–18. Which of the following is a clear indication for MRI during pregnancy?

a. breech presentation in labor
b. suspected appendicidal abscess
c. suspected brain tumor
d. evaluation of epilepsy

46

Critical Care and Trauma

46–1. Which of the following conditions is NOT an indication for invasive hemodynamic monitoring?

a. unexplained pulmonary edema
b. adult respiratory distress syndrome
c. peripartum coronary artery disease
d. "uncomplicated eclampsia"

46–2. Which of the following formulas represents systemic vascular resistance?

a. stroke volume/BSA
b. (MAP-CVP)/CO × 80
c. (MPAP-PCWP)/CO × 80
d. cardiac output/BSA

46–3. Which of the following parameters is used to assess left ventricular end-diastolic filling pressure (i.e., "preload")?

a. central venous pressure
b. pulmonary capillary wedge pressure
c. cardiac index
d. stroke volume

46–4. What two values are needed to construct a left ventricular function curve (i.e., Starling curve)?

a. cardiac output and pulmonary capillary wedge pressure
b. cardiac index and pulmonary vascular resistance

c. stroke index and systemic vascular resistance
d. left ventricular stroke work index and colloid oncotic pressure

46–5. What is ventricular wall tension during systole?

a. preload
b. afterload
c. stroke index
d. cardiac index

46–6. Which of the following is a commonly used agent for reduction in afterload in obstetrical patients?

a. sodium nitroprusside
b. hydralazine
c. lasix
d. propranolol

46–7. Which of the following agents is NOT utilized to improve myocardial contractility (i.e., inotropic state of the heart)?

a. dopamine
b. dobutamine
c. propranolol
d. isoproterenol

46–8. What is the most common complication from pulmonary artery catheterization?

   a. premature ventricular contractions
   b. arterial puncture
   c. pulmonary infarction
   d. pneumothorax

46–9. What is the mortality rate for acute respiratory failure in pregnant women?

   a. <1%
   b. 10%
   c. 25%
   d. 50%

46–10. Which of the following is NOT a criterion for diagnosing the adult respiratory distress syndrome?

   a. $PO_2 < 50$ mm Hg with $FiO_2 > 0.6$
   b. pulmonary capillary wedge pressure $\leq$ 12 mm Hg
   c. functional residual capacity reduced
   d. respiratory rate $\geq$ 15 per min

46–11. How much oxygen is carried by each gram of hemoglobin at 90 percent saturation?

   a. 0.5 mL
   b. 1.25 mL
   c. 2.5 mL
   d. 5.0 mL

46–12. What is the minimum PO_2 necessary to maintain a 90 percent oxyhemoglobin saturation?

   a. 60 mm Hg
   b. 70 mm Hg
   c. 80 mm Hg
   d. 90 mm Hg

46–13. Which of the following is NOT associated with a rightward shift in the oxyhemoglobin dissociation curve (i.e., decreased hemoglobin affinity for oxygen and increased tissue–capillary interchange)?

   a. hypercapnea
   b. metabolic acidosis
   c. increased temperature
   d. decreased 2,3-diphosphoglycerate

46–14. Which of the following colloid oncotic pressures is characteristic of severe preeclampsia during the postpartum period?

   a. 30 mm Hg
   b. 25 mm Hg
   c. 18 mm Hg
   d. 14 mm Hg

46–15. Under normal circumstances, what is the usual colloid oncotic pressure/wedge pressure gradient?

   a. 2 mm Hg
   b. 4 mm Hg
   c. 6 mm Hg
   d. $\geq$8 mm Hg

46–16. Which of the following group of bacteria is most likely to be associated with septic shock?

   a. *Enterobacteriaceae*
   b. anaerobic streptococci
   c. *Bacteroides* species
   d. *Clostridium* species

46–17. Which of the following organisms produces an endotoxin as opposed to an exotoxin?

   a. *Pseudomonas aeruginosa*
   b. *Staphylococcus aureus*
   c. group A streptococcus
   d. *Escherichia coli*

46–18. Which of the following is directly released after gram-negative bacteria are lysed?

   a. complement
   b. kinins
   c. lipopolysaccharide
   d. tumor necrosis factor

46–19. Which dose of dopamine causes α-receptor stimulation (i.e., increased vascular resistance and blood pressure)?

   a. <2 µg/kg
   b. 5 to 10 µg/kg
   c. 10 to 20 µg/kg
   d. 50 to 60 µg/kg

46–20. What percentage of major maternal injuries are associated with traumatic placental abruptions?

    a. 1 to 6
    b. 15
    c. 33
    d. 50

46–21. Approximately what percentage of women with a traumatic placental abruption will have clinically significant hypofibrinogenemia?

    a. 5
    b. 25
    c. 33
    d. 66

46–22. Which of the following signs is most useful in predicting the absence of a placental abruption following trauma?

    a. absence of uterine contractions
    b. absence of bleeding
    c. presence of normal fetal heart tones
    d. absence of tense, painful uterus

46–23. What is the incidence of maternal visceral injuries secondary to penetrating trauma?

    a. 20%
    b. 50%
    c. 75%
    d. nearly 100%

46–24. What is the best management of a pregnant woman at 30 weeks' gestation with burns over 60 percent of her body?

    a. continuous electronic monitoring of the fetus
    b. weekly biophysical profiles
    c. immediate delivery
    d. twice weekly contraction stress tests

Cardiovascular Diseases

47–1. What is the incidence of heart disease in pregnancy?

    a. 0.1%
    b. 1.0%
    c. 5.0%
    d. 10.0%

47–2. What causes the majority of heart disease in pregnancy?

    a. idiopathic cardiomyopathy
    b. constrictive pericarditis
    c. hypertension
    d. congenital heart lesions

47–3. What is the major contributor to cardiac output in pregnancy?

    a. stroke volume
    b. heart rate
    c. blood volume
    d. vascular resistance

47–4. Which of the following symptoms in pregnancy is suggestive of heart disease?

    a. tachycardia
    b. tachypnea
    c. syncope with exertion
    d. peripheral edema

47–5. Which of the following clinical findings warrants an evaluation for underlying heart disease?

    a. systolic murmur, grade II/VI
    b. 1+ peripheral edema
    c. hypertension
    d. persistent neck vein distention

47–6. What is the radiation dosage (maximum) expected with thallium^{201} studies?

    a. 50 mrad
    b. 250 mrad
    c. 610 mrad
    d. 1100 mrad

47–7. Based on echocardiography, which of the following is a common finding in normal pregnancy?

    a. tricuspid regurgitation
    b. mitral regurgitation
    c. aortic stenosis
    d. pulmonary stenosis

47–8. What is the New York Heart Association classification of a woman comfortable at rest but with dyspnea and fatigue during normal activities?

    a. I
    b. II
    c. III
    d. IV

47–9. According to ACOG classification, which of the following heart lesions is associated with the greatest maternal mortality?

    a. patent ductus arteriosus
    b. aortic coarctation with valvular involvement
    c. corrected tetralogy of Fallot
    d. mitral stenosis with atrial fibrillation

47–10. In a woman who is New York Heart Association class I or II, maternal mortality is low, but congestive heart failure during pregnancy has been reported to approach what percentage?

    a. 5
    b. 10
    c. 20
    d. 40

47–11. What is the first warning sign of cardiac failure?

    a. persistent rales at lung base
    b. dyspnea on exertion
    c. hemoptysis
    d. progressive edema

47–12. Which of the following anesthetic techniques is contraindicated in a woman with pulmonary hypertension?

    a. intravenous analgesia
    b. pudendal block
    c. spinal block
    d. general anesthesia

47–13. What is the maternal mortality rate for NYHC III or IV?

    a. 1%
    b. 2 to 3%
    c. 4 to 7%
    d. 10 to 12%

47–14. Which of the following is NOT part of the management of intrapartum heart failure?

    a. Trendelenburg position
    b. morphine
    c. oxygen
    d. furosemide

47–15. What are the effects of pregnancy on long-term prognosis of rheumatic heart disease?

    a. no effect on course
    b. decreases the rate of deterioration
    c. slightly increases the rate of deterioration
    d. markedly increases the rate of deterioration

47–16. Which of the following mechanical valve types is associated with less thromboembolic episodes?

    a. Bjork–Shiley prosthesis
    b. St. Jude medical prosthesis
    c. porcine xenografts
    d. no differences

47–17. Which of the following anticoagulant regimens is recommended during pregnancy in a woman with a mechanical valve?

  a. warfarin orally to maintain partial thromboplastin time two times normal

  b. warfarin orally during the first trimester, then heparin until delivery with partial thromboplastin time maintained at two times normal

  c. heparin intravenously to maintain partial thromboplastin time two times normal

  d. heparin subcutaneously to maintain partial thromboplastin time two times normal

47–18. Which of the following is the fetal response to cardiopulmonary bypass?

  a. persistent late decelerations

  b. bradycardia

  c. tachycardia

  d. repetitive variable decelerations

47–19. Which of the following maternal complications is increased in pregnancies with the previous mitral valvotomy?

  a. heart failure

  b. embolus

  c. cardiac arrest

  d. all of the above

47–20. Which of the following pregnancy complications is increased in women who have undergone mitral valvotomy?

  a. preterm labor

  b. spontaneous abortion

  c. perinatal mortality

  d. none

47–21. Which of the following is true during pregnancy of a woman with a transplanted heart?

  a. does not undergo the normal physiological changes

  b. undergoes the normal physiological changes

  c. has an increased response to normal physiological changes

  d. is at an increased risk of rejection secondary to the stress of pregnancy

47–22. What is the incidence of rheumatic valvular disease in childbearing-aged women?

  a. <0.1%

  b. 0.5 to 1.0%

  c. 2.0 to 4.0%

  d. 10 to 20%

47–23. What valvular lesion causes impediment of blood flow from the left atrium to the left ventricle?

  a. aortic stenosis

  b. aortic regurgitation

  c. mitral stenosis

  d. mitral regurgitation

47–24. What is the surface area of the normal mitral valve?

  a. 1.0 cm^2

  b. 2.5 cm^2

  c. 4.0 cm^2

  d. 5.5 cm^2

47–25. Women with mitral stenosis are at great risk for which condition during labor?

  a. mural thrombosis

  b. myocardial infarction

  c. atrial flutter

  d. rate-related heart failure

47–26. Management of a laboring woman with mitral stenosis should NOT include which of the following?

  a. epidural analgesia

  b. endocarditis prophylaxis

  c. β-blockers to slow heart rate

  d. elective cesarean section

47–27. During pregnancy, what happens to regurgitation associated with the mitral valve?

  a. decreases

  b. remains the same

  c. increases mildly

  d. increases significantly

47–28. What is the size of a normal aortic valve orifice?

  a. <0.5 cm^2

  b. 0.5 to 1.0 cm^2

  c. 2.0 to 3.0 cm^2

  d. >4.0 cm^2

47–29. Management during labor in a woman with symptomatic aortic stenosis should include which of the following?

    a. bacterial endocarditis prophylaxis
    b. avoidance of epidural anesthesia
    c. elective forceps to shorten the second stage of labor
    d. all of the above

47–30. What factor is responsible for improvement in aortic insufficiency and mitral valve incompetence during pregnancy?

    a. increased blood volume
    b. decreased peripheral vascular resistance
    c. increased pulse
    d. all of the above

47–31. Which is the most common atrial septal defect (ASD)?

    a. ostium secundum type
    b. ovale type
    c. ostium primum type
    d. Roger type

47–32. Which of the following is the most common congenital heart defect identified in the newborn period?

    a. patent ductus arteriosus
    b. atrial septal defect
    c. ventricular septal defect
    d. pulmonary stenosis

47–33. In which of the following maternal clinical situations is termination of pregnancy recommended?

    a. aortic stenosis
    b. ventricular septal defect
    c. tetralogy of Fallot, corrected
    d. Eisenmenger syndrome

47–34. Which of the following cardiac lesions is NOT associated with right-to-left shunting of blood?

    a. coarctation of the aorta
    b. tetralogy of Fallot
    c. Ebstein anomaly
    d. transposition of the great vessels

47–35. Which of the following is NOT an associated finding in tetralogy of Fallot?

    a. ventricular septal defect
    b. overriding aorta
    c. right ventricular hypertrophy
    d. pulmonary stenosis

47–36. What is the preferred mode of delivery in a woman with cyanotic heart disease?

    a. vaginal delivery with intravenous sedation for labor
    b. elective cesarean section under general anesthesia
    c. vaginal delivery with epidural analgesia during labor
    d. elective cesarean section under epidural analgesia

47–37. Which of the following is associated with the development of Eisenmenger syndrome?

    a. right-to-left shunting
    b. pulmonary hypertension
    c. pulmonary vascular resistance greater than systemic vascular resistance
    d. all of the above

47–38. What is the etiology of maternal mortality in women with pulmonary hypertension?

    a. right ventricular overload
    b. diminished venous return
    c. pulmonary emboli
    d. mural thrombosis

47–39. In which of the following should women with mitral valve prolapse receive intrapartum bacterial endocarditis prophylaxis?

    a. if there is mitral valve regurgitation
    b. when there is excessive blood loss
    c. if cesarean section is necessary
    b. in all cases

47–40. Which of the following has been identified in women with peripartum heart failure?

    a. superimposed pregnancy-induced hypertension
    b. mitral stenosis
    c. viral myocarditis
    d. all of the above

47–41. What is the incidence of idiopathic cardiomyopathy during pregnancy?

    a. 1 in 3000
    b. 1 in 9000
    c. 1 in 15,000
    d. 1 in 30,000

47–42. What is the hallmark finding in idiopathic cardiomyopathy?

    a. rales
    b. peripheral edema
    c. diastolic murmur
    d. cardiomegaly

47–43. Which of the following is NOT recommended in the antepartum management of idiopathic cardiomyopathy?

    a. heparin
    b. digitalis
    c. angiotensin-converting enzyme inhibitor
    d. furosemide

47–44. Which of the following is a low-risk factor for bacterial endocarditis?

    a. aortic stenosis
    b. atrial septal defect
    c. ventricular septal defect
    d. aortic coarctation

47–45. Which is the predominant organism in parenteral drug abusers with bacterial endocarditis?

    a. *Staphylococcus aureus,* coagulase positive
    b. *Streptococcus pneumoniae*
    c. *Neisseria gonorrhoeae*
    d. *Staphylococcus epidermidis,* coagulase negative

47–46. Which of the following lesions secondary to bacterial endocarditis is difficult to diagnose with echocardiography?

    a. 1-cm lesion on the aortic valve
    b. 0.5-cm lesion on the mitral valve
    c. 0.5-cm lesion on the aortic valve
    d. 1-cm lesion on the tricuspid valve

47–47. According to 1990 guidelines, during which obstetrical procedure are prophylactic antibiotics recommended?

    a. chorionic villus sampling
    b. vaginal delivery in the presence of infection
    c. cesarean section
    d. dilatation and curettage

47–48. Which of the following tachyarrhythmia is the most common in pregnancy?

    a. Wolff-Parkinson-White syndrome
    b. paroxysmal supraventricular tachycardia
    c. ventricular tachycardia
    d. none of the above

47–49. Which condition does NOT place a pregnant woman at increased risk for aortic dissection?

    a. Marfan syndrome
    b. coarctation of the aorta
    c. Noonan syndrome
    d. syphilitic aortitis

47–50. How is the definite diagnosis of aortic dissection made?

    a. chest x-ray
    b. aortic angiography
    c. sonography
    d. magnetic resonance imaging

47–51. How is Marfan syndrome inherited?

    a. autosomal recessive
    b. autosomal dominant
    c. X-linked dominant
    d. polygenic

47–52. The gene defect associated with Marfan syndrome is located on which of the following chromosomes?

    a. 3p
    b. 6q
    c. 15q
    d. 20p

47–53. Which gene is abnormal in Marfan syndrome?

    a. tubulin
    b. connexin
    c. fibrillin
    d. muscularium

47–54. Women are at increased risk for cardiovascular complications with aortic dilatation greater than which of the following?

    a. 20 mm in diameter
    b. 30 mm in diameter
    c. 40 mm in diameter
    d. 50 mm in diameter

47–55. What is the incidence of maternal mortality associated with aortic coarctation?

    a. 1%
    b. 3%
    c. 10%
    d. 30%

47–56. Myocardial infarctions in women without coronary artery disease have been associated with which of the following?

    a. oxytocin induction of labor
    b. prostaglandin gel for cervical ripening
    c. prostaglandin $F_{2\alpha}$ to control atony
    d. prostaglandin E_2 suppositories to induce labor

47–57. Which of the following has NOT been associated with myocardial infarction?

    a. bromocriptine to suppress lactation
    b. prostaglandin E_2 to induce labor
    c. high-dose oxytocin for termination of pregnancy
    d. ergonovine for postpartum hemorrhage

47–58. Concerning myocardial infarction in pregnancy, women are at greatest risk for mortality if the infarction occurs during which of the following periods?

    a. 1st trimester
    b. 2nd trimester
    c. 2 weeks prior to labor
    d. 2 weeks after delivery

47–59. How is the diagnosis of idiopathic hypertrophic subaortic stenosis (IHSS) made?

    a. clinical examination
    b. Doppler echocardiography
    c. computed tomography scan
    d. magnetic resonance imaging

48

Pulmonary Disorders

48–1. What is the incidence of asthma in pregnancy?

    a. 0.1 to 0.4%
    b. 1.0 to 4.0%
    c. 10 to 14%
    d. 20 to 24%

48–2. Which of the following cannot be measured directly?

    a. tidal volume
    b. residual volume

    c. minute ventilation
    d. inspiratory capacity

48–3. Which of the following characterizes functional residual capacity during pregnancy?

    a. decreases by approximately 500 mL
    b. stays unchanged compared with nonpregnant values
    c. increases by about 500 mL
    d. increases by about 1 L

48–4. How much does basal oxygen consumption increase by the second trimester

   a. 5 mL/min
   b. 10 mL/min
   c. 20 mL/min
   d. 100 mL/min

48–5. Which is inflammation of the lung parenchyma distal to the large airways and involving alveolar units?

   a. pneumonia
   b. asthma
   c. bronchopneumonia
   d. sarcoidosis

48–6. Which of the following organisms is the major cause of bacterial pneumonia in otherwise healthy patients?

   a. *Staphylococcus aureus*
   b. *Chlamydia trachomatis*
   c. *Mycoplasma pneumoniae*
   d. *Streptococcus pneumoniae*

48–7. Which of the following is a risk factor for lung colonization with Legionella?

   a. smoking
   b. asthma
   c. ear infection
   d. alcohol

48–8. A 27-year-old woman at 32 weeks' gestation presents complaining of cough, fever, chest pain, and dyspnea. Which of the following tests would be most helpful in making a diagnosis?

   a. complete blood cell count
   b. mycoplasma-specific immunoglobulin G
   c. urinalysis for pneumococcal antigen
   d. chest x-ray

48–9. Which of the following factors is NOT an indication for hospitalization of a woman with pneumonia?

   a. altered mental status
   b. hypertension
   c. hypothermia
   d. respiratory rate >30/min

48–10. What is first-line therapy in a pregnant woman with community-acquired pneumonia?

   a. dicloxicillin
   b. clindamycin
   c. ampicillin
   d. erythromycin

48–11. Pneumococcal vaccine should be given for which of the following conditions?

   a. sickle cell disease
   b. gestational diabetes
   c. pregnancy-induced hypertension
   d. all pregnancies

48–12. Which of the following perinatal complications is associated with bacterial pneumonia?

   a. fetal growth retardation
   b. preterm labor
   c. persistent fetal circulation
   d. cerebral palsy

48–13. Pregnant women with which finding should be vaccinated against influenza?

   a. sickle cell trait
   b. hyperthyroidism
   c. insulin-dependent diabetes
   d. asymptomatic bacteriuria

48–14. What is the treatment of choice for early onset influenza in pregnancy?

   a. retrovir
   b. amantadine
   c. acyclovir
   d. ganciclovir

48–15. Primary infection of varicella may lead to pneumonia in what percentage of adults?

   a. 10
   b. 20
   c. 30
   d. 40

48–16. In a seronegative individual exposed to active infection, what is the attack rate for varicella?

   a. 30%
   b. 50%
   c. 70%
   d. 90%

48–17. Which of the following agents lowers the mortality in varicella pneumonia?

    a. acyclovir
    b. varicella zoster immunoglobulin
    c. gamma globulin
    d. all of the above

48–18. What is the best management for a susceptible pregnant woman exposed to varicella less than 96 hours?

    a. varicella isoimmunization IM
    b. varivax
    c. acyclovir prophylaxis
    d. expectant management/observation

48–19. What is the mortality of varicella pneumonia during pregnancy?

    a. 5%
    b. 15%
    c. 35%
    d. 90%

48–20. Chemical pneumonitis from aspiration of gastric contents is the consequence of which of the following?

    a. gastrin
    b. bradykinin
    c. hydrochloric acid
    d. bicitric acid

48–21. Which of the following treatment regimens is effective for *Pneumocystis carinii* pneumonia?

    a. ampicillin
    b. erythromycin
    c. trimethoprim–sulfamethoxazole
    d. azithromycin

48–22. In which of the following HIV-positive patients is aerosolized pentamidine or oral trimethoprim–sulfamethoxazole recommended prophylactically to prevent pneumocystis infection?

    a. CD4 count < 200/mL
    b. CD4 count < 500/mL
    c. CD4 count < 750/mL
    d. all HIV-positive women

48–23. Which of the following may have stimulatory effects on estradiol-17β?

    a. coccidioidomycosis
    b. histoplasmosis
    c. blastomycosis
    d. sarcoidosis

48–24. What percentage of the general population has asthma?

    a. 0.5 to 1.5
    b. 3.0 to 4.0
    c. 6.0 to 8.0
    d. 10.0 to 12.0

48–25. What proportion of asthmatics can expect worsening of disease during pregnancy?

    a. none
    b. one-fourth
    c. one-third
    d. one-half

48–26. Which of the following pregnancy complications is NOT increased in asthmatics?

    a. preterm labor
    b. perinatal mortality
    c. low-birthweight infants
    d. congenital anomalies

48–27. If a pregnant asthmatic requires mechanical ventilation, the mortality rate approaches what level?

    a. 20%
    b. 40%
    c. 60%
    d. 80%

48–28. Which of the following is a primary mediator of asthma?

    a. thromboxanes
    b. leukotrienes
    c. prostaglandins
    d. histamines

48–29. Which of the following findings is associated with the "danger zone" stage of asthma?

    a. pO_2 normal; pCO_2 decreased; pH increased
    b. pO_2 normal; pCO_2 increased; pH normal

c. pO_2 decreased; pCO_2 normal; pH normal

d. pO_2 decreased; pCO_2 decreased; pH increased

48–30. Which of the FEV_1 presented, as percentage of predicted values, is associated with respiratory acidosis (stage 4 asthma)?

a. <35
b. 35 to 49
c. 50 to 64
d. 65 to 80

48–31. For which reason is the pregnant asthmatic more likely to develop hypoxia?

a. increased residual volume
b. decreased function residual capacity
c. decreased tidal volume
d. increased inspiratory capacity

48–32. Which signs point to a potentially fatal asthmatic attack?

a. use of accessory muscles, labored breathing
b. central cyanosis, labored breathing
c. use of accessory muscles, prolonged expiration
d. central cyanosis, altered consciousness

48–33. Which of the following tests is most useful in monitoring airway obstruction?

a. chest x-ray
b. arterial blood gas
c. FEV_1 (forced expiratory volume in 1 second)
d. pulse oximeter

48–34. Which is the first-line therapy for acute asthma?

a. antibiotics
b. β-adrenergic agonist
c. methylxanthines
d. cromolyn sodium

48–35. Which of the following agents is used to stabilize mast cell membranes?

a. theophylline
b. cromolyn sulfate
c. corticosteroids
d. epinephrine

48–36. Which of the following analgesics is a non-histamine-releasing narcotic and therefore should be used for asthmatics?

a. morphine
b. meperidine
c. fentanyl
d. codeine

48–37. Which agent should be used to treat postpartum hemorrhage in an asthmatic?

a. oxytocin
b. prostaglandin $F_{2\alpha}$
c. 15-methyl $PGF_{2\alpha}$
d. any of the above

48–38. In which of the following locations is a pulmonary embolus unlikely to have originated?

a. superficial thigh veins
b. deep veins—leg
c. deep veins—thigh
d. deep veins—pelvis

48–39. What is the treatment for superficial thrombophlebitis?

a. analgesia and coumarin
b. analgesia and rest
c. "minidose" heparin
d. full anticoagulation

48–40. Which of the following deficiencies is NOT associated with increased incidence of thromboembolic complications?

a. protein M
b. protein S
c. protein C
d. antithrombin III

48–41. Phlegmasia alba dolens is clinically suspected in which of the following situations?

a. There is abrupt onset of leg pain and edema.
b. Edema of both lower extremities exists.
c. Red hot lower extremity is noted.
d. None of the above apply.

48–42. What is the most accurate method to diagnose deep venous thrombosis?

    a. impedance plethysmography
    b. real-time β-mode ultrasonography
    c. venography
    d. color Doppler ultrasonography

48–43. What is the approximate incidence of pulmonary embolism associated with pregnancy?

    a. 1 in 70 deliveries
    b. 1 in 700 deliveries
    c. 1 in 7000 deliveries
    d. 1 in 70,000 deliveries

48–44. What percentage of patients with pulmonary embolus have the classic triad of hemoptysis, dyspnea, and pleuritic chest pain?

    a. 20
    b. 40
    c. 60
    d. 80

48–45. A negative ventilation–perfusion scan is associated with pulmonary embolism in what percentage of patients?

    a. <1
    b. 2 to 4
    c. 8 to 10
    d. >15

48–46. What is the radiation exposure to the fetus from pulmonary angiography?

    a. 6 to 18 mrad
    b. 70 to 80 mrad
    c. 220 to 370 mrad
    d. 530 to 618 mrad

48–47. When continuous intravenous heparin is compared with intermittent subcutaneous heparin for anticoagulation, which of the following is likely?

    a. Initial anticoagulation with intravenous heparin is suboptimal.
    b. Recurrent thromboembolism is more commonly associated with subcutaneous heparin.

    c. Intravenous heparin is associated with excessively prolonged bleeding times.
    d. There is no difference between the two regimens.

48–48. In general, for "full" anticoagulation, what should the total daily dose of heparin be?

    a. 5 to 10,000 U
    b. 15 to 20,000 U
    c. 24 to 28,000 U
    d. 30 to 40,000 U

48–49. In giving heparin subcutaneously every 12 hours, when should the activated partial thromboplastin time be checked?

    a. 2 hours after last dose
    b. 4 hours after last dose
    c. 6 hours after last dose
    d. immediately prior to next dose

48–50. A major side effect of heparin is osteoporosis. This is more likely to occur in which situation listed below?

    a. less than 20,000 units are given per day for a short time
    b. treatment exceeds 6 months
    c. more than 20,000 units per day are given for 3 months
    d. more than 20,000 units per day are given for 6 months

48–51. What is the major risk with low-dose heparin?

    a. hemorrhage
    b. thrombosis
    c. osteoporosis
    d. thrombocytopenia

48–52. Which of the following is NOT a congenital malformation associated with warfarin?

    a. ophthalmological abnormality
    b. retarded development
    c. nasal hypoplasia
    d. limb hypoplasia

48–53. Which of the following is given to reverse the anticoagulation effects of warfarin within 8 hours?

    a. protamine sulfate intravenously
    b. vitamin D

c. vitamin E

d. vitamin K 10 mg intravenously

48–54. How should a woman with deep venous thrombosis in a previous pregnancy be managed in a current pregnancy?

a. careful observation

b. minidose subcutaneous heparin

c. full prophylactic subcutaneous heparin

d. low-dose aspirin

48–55. Which of the following groups is NOT particularly at risk for tuberculosis?

a. those who are pregnant

b. the elderly

c. the urban poor

d. minorities

48–56. How should nonpregnant patients who are tuberculin-positive but x-ray negative be treated?

a. rifampin 10 mg/kg daily for 4 months

b. streptomycin for 12 months

c. isoniazid 300 mg daily for 12 months

d. pyridoxine for 12 months

48–57. How should a pregnant woman who is tuberculin-positive but x-ray negative be managed?

a. rifampin 10 mg/kg daily for 12 months

b. isoniazid 300 mg daily for 12 months

c. ethambutol for 12 months

d. observation and treatment after delivery

48–58. Which of the following antituberculosis agents is associated with severe deafness if given to a pregnant woman?

a. streptomycin

b. isoniazid

c. rifampin

d. ethambutol

48–59. What of the following x-ray findings is the hallmark of sarcoidosis?

a. mediastinal widening

b. diffuse infiltrates

c. patchy infiltrates

d. interstitial pneumonitis

48–60. How is symptomatic severe pulmonary sarcoidosis treated?

a. betamethasone 12 mg IM every day

b. decadron 6 mg orally twice a day

c. prednisone 1 mg/kg/day

d. cyclophosphamide 1 mg/kg/day

48–61. Which of the following electrolyte patterns in sweat is associated with cystic fibrosis?

a. ↑ sodium; ↓ potassium; ↑ chloride

b. ↑ sodium; ↑ potassium; ↓ chloride

c. ↑ sodium; ↓ potassium; ↓ chloride

d. ↑ sodium; ↑ potassium; ↑ chloride

48–62. Lung function in women with cystic fibrosis is improved by using which of the following to decrease the viscosity of sputum?

a. recombinant human DNase

b. acetylcysteine mist

c. bronchodilators

d. diuretics

$\boxed{49}$

Renal and Urinary Tract Disorders

49–1. During pregnancy, effective renal plasma flow is increased by what percentage?

   a. 5
   b. 10
   c. 20
   d. 40

49–2. What is the cutoff for significant proteinuria during pregnancy?

   a. 50 mg/day
   b. 100 mg/day
   c. 200 mg/day
   d. 500 mg/day

49–3. What is the average excretion of albumin during pregnancy?

   a. <50 mg
   b. 100 mg
   c. 200 mg
   d. 500 mg

49–4. What is postural (orthostatic) proteinuria?

   a. abnormal urine protein when patient is ambulatory
   b. abnormal urine protein secondary to mild renal disease
   c. abnormal urine protein due to bacteriuria
   d. abnormal urine protein at nighttime in a patient with hypertension

49–5. Which of the following enhances the virulence of *E. coli*?

   a. glycoprotein receptors
   b. P-fimbriae
   c. exotoxins
   d. nuclear pili

49–6. Which of the following is most likely to be associated with covert bacteriuria?

   a. age < 20 years
   b. hypertension
   c. sickle cell trait
   d. lupus

49–7. What is the adverse pregnancy outcome associated with asymptomatic bacteriuria?

   a. low-birthweight infant
   b. preterm delivery
   c. acute antepartum pyelonephritis
   d. pregnancy-induced hypertension

49–8. What is the most likely diagnosis in a woman with frequency, urgency, pyuria, dysuria, and a sterile urine culture?

   a. *E. coli* cystitis
   b. group B streptococcus cystitis
   c. *Chlamydia trachomatis* urethritis
   d. *N. gonorrhoeae* urethritis

49–9. What is the most common serious medical complication of pregnancy?

   a. cystitis
   b. pneumonia
   c. pancreatitis
   d. pyelonephritis

49–10. Of the bacteria that cause renal infection, what is the incidence of P-fimbriae?

   a. 10%
   b. 35%
   c. 70%
   d. >80%

49–11. What organism is associated with antepartum pyelonephritis?

a. *Listeria monocytogenes*
b. *Klebsiella pneumoniae*
c. *Pseudomonas*
d. *Peptostreptococcus*

49–12. Which of the following is NOT included in the differential diagnosis for pyelonephritis?

a. chorioamnionitis
b. labor
c. pneumonia
d. abruptio placenta

49–13. What causes the large temperature swings (i.e.,"hypothalamic instability") in pyelonephritis?

a. cytokines
b. interferons
c. endorphins
d. exotoxins

49–14. What percentage of women with acute antepartum pyelonephritis have bacteremia?

a. 7.5
b. 15.0
c. 22.5
d. 30.0

49–15. Which of the following causes alveolar injury and hence respiratory insufficiency in women with pyelonephritis?

a. prostaglandins
b. cytokines
c. interferons
d. endotoxins

49–16. What is the initial drug of choice for the treatment of pyelonephritis in pregnancy?

a. ampicillin
b. cephalosporin
c. an aminoglycoside
d. empirical

49–17. What percentage of renal stones are radiopaque?

a. 60
b. 70
c. 80
d. 90

49–18. An 18-year-old nulliparous black woman has been on antibiotics for 4 days for pyelonephritis. She continues to have fever ranging from 38.9 to 39.6°C. Workup reveals a right ureteral obstruction secondary to calculi. What is the next most appropriate step in her management?

a. Change her antibiotics.
b. Continue the present antibiotics for at least 7 days.
c. Pass a double-J ureteral stent.
d. Perform a percutaneous nephrostomy.

49–19. What is the composition of the majority of renal stones?

a. struvite
b. calcium salts
c. uric acid
d. magnesium salts

49–20. What is the most common presenting symptom of renal stones in pregnant women?

a. flank pain
b. abdominal pain
c. hematuria
d. infection

49–21. Which of the following is NOT one of the five major glomerulopathic syndromes?

a. rapidly progressive glomerulonephritis
b. chronic pyelonephritis
c. nephrotic syndrome
d. acute glomerulonephritis

49–22. Which of the following lists signs and symptoms of acute glomerulonephritis?

a. hematuria, proteinuria, edema, and hypertension
b. proteinuria and hypertension but no edema
c. hematuria, hypotension, and proteinuria
d. proteinuria, hypotension, and edema

49–23. Which of the following is NOT a fetal effect of glomerulonephritis?

a. fetal loss
b. fetal growth retardation
c. preterm birth
d. fetal intraventricular hemorrhage

49–24. What is the incidence of hypertension in pregnancy in women with glomerulonephritis?

a. 10%
b. 25%
c. 50%
d. 75%

49–25. What percentage of women with primary glomerulonephritis have worsening proteinuria?

a. 20
b. 40
c. 60
d. 80

49–26. Which of the following is NOT associated with a poor perinatal prognosis in parturients with glomerulonephritis?

a. impaired renal function
b. severe hypertension
c. anemia
d. proteinuria greater than 5 g/24 hr

49–27. What are the characteristics of nephrotic syndrome?

a. proteinuria > 300 mg/day, hyperlipidemia, and edema
b. proteinuria > 300 mg/day and hypolipidemia
c. proteinuria > 3000 mg/day, hyperlipidemia, and edema
d. proteinuria > 3000 mg/day and hypolipidemia

49–28. Which of the following is NOT a cause of nephrotic syndrome?

a. IgA nephropathy
b. sarcoidosis
c. poststreptococcal glomerulonephritis
d. heroin use

49–29. Successful pregnancy outcomes can be anticipated in women with nephrosis in which of the following circumstances?

a. Woman is normotensive.
b. Renal insufficiency is moderate.
c. Proteinuria is less than 5 g/day.
d. Hypertension is controlled with blood pressure medications.

49–30. What is the significance of proteinuria if it antedates pregnancy?

a. It is benign.
b. It is associated with anemia.
c. Hypertension is not increased.
d. Preterm delivery is not increased.

49–31. Which describes the mechanism of inheritance in adult polycystic kidney disease?

a. sporadic
b. X-linked recessive
c. autosomal recessive
d. autosomal dominant

49–32. Polycystic kidney disease is linked to the α-hemoglobin gene complex on the short arm of which chromosome?

a. 1
b. 11
c. 16
d. X

49–33. Which of the following is NOT a symptom of polycystic kidney disease?

a. flank pain
b. nocturia
c. fever
d. malaise

49–34. Which of the following is NOT associated with polycystic kidneys?

a. hepatic cysts
b. cardiac valvular lesions
c. diverticulosis
d. Berry aneurysm

49–35. What is the adverse effect of pregnancy on women with polycystic kidney disease?

a. increased spontaneous abortion
b. increased stillbirths

c. increased symptomatic urinary infection

d. no adverse effect

49–36. What is the most common cause of end-stage renal disease?

a. diabetes
b. hypertension
c. glomerulonephritis
d. polycystic kidney disease

49–37. What is the average blood volume expansion in pregnant women with severe renal insufficiency?

a. 10%
b. 25%
c. 35%
d. 45%

49–38. Which of the following is NOT associated with pregnancies in women with chronic renal insufficiency?

a. anemia
b. hypertension
c. hypercalcemia
d. preeclampsia

49–39. Which of the following is a major side effect from recombinant erythropoietin use in pregnancy?

a. hyperviscosity
b. hypertension
c. human immunodeficiency viral transmission
d. worsening renal function

49–40. In pregnancies complicated by severe renal insufficiency, pregnancy itself causes which of the following?

a. accelerated renal insufficiency
b. complete resolution of renal insufficiency
c. partial resolution of renal insufficiency
d. no appreciable change in renal function

49–41. Which of the following is NOT included in the differential diagnosis of renal transplant rejection during pregnancy?

a. pyelonephritis
b. preeclampsia
c. respiratory distress syndrome
d. recurrent glomerulonephropathy

49–42. Which of the following is most helpful in making the diagnosis of renal transplant rejection during pregnancy?

a. renal biopsy
b. clinical symptoms
c. urinalysis
d. renal vein laboratory studies

49–43. Which of the following medications is an FDA Category D drug?

a. prednisone
b. azathioprine
c. cyclosporine
d. erythropoietin

49–44. Which of the following tests is useful for monitoring the toxic effects of azathioprine?

a. serum hepatic enzymes
b. urinalysis for protein
c. serum creatinine
d. complete blood count, including platelets

49–45. What percentage of pregnancies in women on chronic hemodialysis result in a live birth?

a. 10
b. 25
c. 50
d. 75

49–46. Which of the following laboratory values represent prerenal azotemia?

a. urine to plasma creatinine > 10; urine to plasma osmolality < 1.0
b. urine to plasma creatinine > 10; urine to plasma osmolality > 1.5
c. urine to plasma creatinine > 20; urine to plasma osmolality < 1.0
d. urine to plasma creatinine > 20; urine to plasma osmolality > 1.5

49–47. What is the amount of urinary sodium in patients with prerenal azotemia?

    a. <1 mEq/L
    b. <5 mEq/L
    c. <20 mEq/L
    d. >50 mEq/L

49–48. Which of the following pregnancy complications is associated with renal cortical necrosis?

    a. eclampsia
    b. placenta abruption
    c. endotoxin-induced shock
    d. placenta previa

50

Gastrointestinal Disorders

50–1. What is the incidence of laparotomy during pregnancy?

    a. 1 in 240
    b. 1 in 500
    c. 1 in 1000
    d. 1 in 5000

50–2. Why does total parenteral nutrition require catheterization of the jugular or subclavian vein?

    a. Thromboembolism occurs if given in a smaller vein.
    b. The solution is hyperosmolar and needs to be diluted in a high-flow system.
    c. Essential fatty acids block smaller veins.
    d. The potassium content causes sclerosis of the smaller veins.

50–3. Which of the following findings would be expected in women with hyperemesis gravidarum?

    a. hematocrit < 30 vol%
    b. creatinine 0.3 mg/dL

    c. ALT 86 IU/L
    d. K+ 5.8 mEq/L

50–4. Which of the following antiemetics is an FDA Category B drug?

    a. metoclopramide
    b. promethazine
    c. chlorpromazine
    d. prochlorperazine

50–5. What is the etiology of reflux esophagitis in pregnancy?

    a. constriction of upper esophageal sphincter
    b. relaxation of upper esophageal sphincter
    c. constriction of lower esophageal sphincter
    d. relaxation of lower esophageal sphincter

50–6. Diaphragmatic hernias are herniations of abdominal contents through which foramen?

    a. Bochdalek
    b. oavale
    c. magnum
    d. Morgan

50–7. Which of the following is a motor disorder of esophageal smooth muscle?

    a. diaphragmatic hernia
    b. hiatal hernia
    c. reflux esophagitis
    d. achalasia

50–8. Which of the following treatments is NOT indicated in the management of achalasia?

    a. soft foods
    b. anticholinergic drugs
    c. pneumatic dilation
    d. hyperalimentation

50–9. Which organism is associated with peptic ulcer disease?

    a. *Heliobacter stomachi*
    b. *Heliobacter pylori*
    c. *Heliobacter acidi*
    d. *Heliobacter gastrecti*

50–10. Which of the following is associated with normal pregnancy?

    a. decreased mucus secretion
    b. increased gastric secretion
    c. decreased gastric motility
    d. constriction of lower esophageal sphincter

50–11. The majority of pregnancies with upper gastrointestinal bleeding have which of the following?

    a. Boerhaave syndrome
    b. stomach cancer
    c. Mallory–Weiss tears
    d. peptic ulceration

50–12. Which of the following is a dangerous complication associated with ulcerative colitis?

    a. toxic megacolon
    b. bloody diarrhea

    c. arthritis
    d. erythema nodosum

50–13. Which of the following HLA haplotypes is associated with ulcerative colitis?

    a. HLA-BW 35
    b. HLA-A2
    c. HLA-B3
    d. HLA-A16

50–14. What is the most likely course for ulcerative colitis that is quiescent at the beginning of gestation?

    a. no activation of disease during pregnancy
    b. active disease during pregnancy in 33%
    c. active disease during pregnancy in 67%
    d. active disease during pregnancy in 100%

50–15. What is the most common long-term complication in a woman who has had a colectomy with mucosal proctectomy and ileal pouch-anal anastomosis?

    a. pouchitis
    b. large bowel obstruction
    c. proctitis
    d. fistula formation

50–16. What is the most common symptom associated with bowel obstruction?

    a. nausea
    b. vomiting
    c. abdominal pain
    d. diarrhea

50–17. What is the cause of pseudo-obstruction of the colon (Ogilvie syndrome)?

    a. pelvic adhesions
    b. impacted stool
    c. adynamic colonic ileus
    d. medications used postpartum

50–18. Which of the following is NOT in the differential diagnosis of appendicitis in pregnancy?

    a. Crohn's disease
    b. placental abruption
    c. pyelonephritis
    d. pneumonia

50–19. Which of the following complications is associated with ruptured appendix and peritonitis?

   a. fetal growth restriction
   b. oligohydramnios
   c. chorioamnionitis
   d. preterm birth

50–20. Which of the following infectious agents is NOT associated with acute colitis in pregnancy?

   a. *E. coli*
   b. *Campylobacter* sp.
   c. *Shigella* sp.
   d. *Hemophilus* sp.

50–21. What happens to cholesterol during normal pregnancy?

   a. remains unchanged
   b. doubles
   c. quadruples
   d. decreases by one half

50–22. Which of the following serum protein concentrations is decreased during pregnancy?

   a. albumin
   b. globulin
   c. ceruloplasmin
   d. transferrin

50–23. What is the major histological lesion of intrahepatic cholestasis?

   a. centrilobular bile staining
   b. mesenchymal proliferation
   c. periportal necrosis
   d. centrilobular necrosis

50–24. How is intrahepatic cholestasis of pregnancy inherited?

   a. multifactorial
   b. X-linked recessive
   c. autosomal recessive
   d. autosomal dominant

50–25. What is the pathogenesis of intrahepatic cholestasis?

   a. increase in human placental lactogen
   b. increase in human chorionic gonadotropin

   c. increase in estrogen
   d. increase in progesterone

50–26. Which of the following is appropriate in the management of intrahepatic cholestasis?

   a. azathioprine
   b. antihistamines
   c. ampicillin
   d. vitamin A

50–27. Which of the following is NOT an adverse pregnancy outcome associated with intrahepatic cholestasis?

   a. abruptio placenta
   b. preterm birth
   c. stillbirth
   d. postpartum hemorrhage

50–28. What is the prominent histologic abnormality associated with acute fatty liver of pregnancy?

   a. intranuclear fat
   b. microvesicular fat
   c. massive hepatocellular necrosis
   d. all of the above

50–29. What is the major symptom in pregnancy complicated by acute fatty liver?

   a. malaise
   b. anorexia
   c. nausea
   d. vomiting

50–30. What is the etiology of diabetes insipidus in pregnancies complicated by acute fatty liver?

   a. excessive levels of oxytocin
   b. elevated vasopressinase concentrations
   c. fatty deposits in supraoptic nuclei
   d. decreased blood flow to posterior pituitary

50–31. What percentage of the liver's blood supply comes from the hepatic artery?

   a. 10
   b. 25
   c. 33
   d. 50

50–32. What is the most common serious liver disease in pregnancy?

    a. intrahepatic cholestasia
    b. hepatitis
    c. preeclampsia
    d. acute fatty liver

50–33. What is the frequency of chronic hepatitis B following acute disease?

    a. <1%
    b. 5 to 10%
    c. 20 to 25%
    d. 40 to 50%

50–34. What is the incubation period for hepatitis A?

    a. 3 to 5 days
    b. 2 to 7 weeks
    c. 10 to 12 weeks
    d. >20 weeks

50–35. Which of the following hepatitis panels is associated with acute hepatitis A and chronic hepatitis B?

	HBsAg	Anti-HAV IgM	Anti-HBc IgM
a.	−	+	−
b.	+	+	+
c.	+	+	−
d.	+	−	+

50–36. Which of the following is recommended for a pregnant woman exposed to hepatitis A?

    a. gamma globulin
    b. hepatitis A immunoglobulin
    c. hepatitis B immunoglobulin (HBIG)
    d. HBIG plus gamma globulin

50–37. Which of the following is a DNA virus?

    a. hepatitis A
    b. hepatitis B
    c. hepatitis C
    d. delta hepatitis

50–38. What percentage of hepatitis B-infected infants develop chronic infection?

    a. <1
    b. 5 to 10
    c. 20 to 30
    d. 70 to 90

50–39. What is the first virological marker for hepatitis B?

    a. HBeAg
    c. HBcAg
    c. HBsAg
    d. HB dane Ag

50–40. What is the significance of the e antigen of hepatitis B virus?

    a. viral shedding in the feces
    b. noninfectivity
    c. number of circulating virus particles
    d. chronic carrier state

50–41. How should infants delivered to chronic hepatitis B carriers be treated?

    a. isolated from their mothers
    b. treated with HBIG
    c. vaccinated with recombinant vaccine
    d. given HBIG and recombinant vaccine

50–42. When is the antibody first detected in the majority of patients with hepatitis C?

    a. at 3 weeks
    b. at 9 weeks
    c. at 15 weeks
    d. at 1 year

50–43. What is the incidence of persistent hepatitis C infection that progresses to cirrhosis within 10 years?

    a. 5%
    b. 10%
    c. 20%
    d. 50%

50–44. Which of the following agents may be effective or beneficial in producing remission in one-half of chronic hepatitis B carriers?

    a. corticosteroids
    b. azathioprine
    c. interferon-α
    d. interleukin-2

50–45. What is the most common cause of cirrhosis in young women?

    a. alcohol
    b. hepatitis
    c. illicit drug use
    d. prescribed drugs

50–46. What is the normal portal vein pressure?

　　a. <5 mm Hg
　　b. 10 to 15 mm Hg
　　c. 30 to 40 mm Hg
　　d. 60 to 80 mm Hg

50–47. What is the treatment of choice for acetaminophen overdosage?

　　a. *N*-acetylcysteine
　　b. glutathione
　　c. emesis induced with charcoal
　　d. aggressive fluids containing sodium bicarbonate

50–48. What is the most common pregnancy complication in women with liver transplants?

　　a. anemia
　　b. hypertension
　　c. preterm delivery
　　d. psychosis

50–49. What is the major component of gallstones?

　　a. cholesterol
　　b. calcium
　　c. bile acids
　　d. struvite

50–50. What is the cause of decreased gallbladder motility?

　　a. estrogen
　　b. progesterone
　　c. cholecystokinin
　　d. relaxin

50–51. Which of the following is NOT a nonsurgical approach for gallstone disease?

　　a. chenodeoxycholic acid
　　b. dietary changes
　　c. intragallbladder methyl terbutyl ether
　　d. extracorporeal shock wave lithotripsy

50–52. Which of the following is relatively contraindicated in pregnancy for the management of gallstones?

　　a. laparoscopic cholecystectomy
　　b. endoscopic retrograde cholangiopancreatography

　　c. laparotomy at 12 weeks' gestation
　　d. none of the above

50–53. Which of the following is NOT a cause of pancreatitis in pregnancy?

　　a. trauma
　　b. hypotriglyceridemia
　　c. alcoholism
　　d. gallstones

50–54. Which of the following portends a bad prognosis in women with pancreatitis?

　　a. twin gestation
　　b. hypercalcemia
　　c. shock
　　d. dehydration

50–55. Which of the following is NOT a complication of pancreatitis?

　　a. abscess
　　b. pseudocyst
　　c. phlegmon
　　d. bowel obstruction

50–56. Which symptom confirms the diagnosis of pancreatitis?

　　a. leukocytosis
　　b. serum amylase three times normal
　　c. low serum lipase
　　d. hypocalcemia

50–57. What percentage of adults are obese?

　　a. 12%
　　b. 25%
　　c. 33%
　　d. 40%

50–58. Which of the following is the most common problem identified in obese as compared to nonobese women?

　　a. hypertension
　　b. postterm pregnancy
　　c. macrosomia
　　d. shoulder dystocia

51

Hematological Disorders

51–1. How much does the blood volume expand during normal pregnancy?

   a. 25%
   b. 50%
   c. 75%
   d. 100%

51–2. What are the total iron requirements for the mother and fetus during a normal pregnancy?

   a. 100 mg
   b. 300 mg
   c. 1000 mg
   d. 3000 mg

51–3. What is the cutoff for hemoglobin concentration for defining anemia during pregnancy?

   a. <8 g/dL
   b. <10 g/dL
   c. <12 g/dL
   d. <14 g/dL

51–4. What causes the increased erythrocyte sedimentation rate in pregnancy?

   a. inflammatory response
   b. induced cytokine
   c. immunological rejection
   d. hyperfibrinogenemia

51–5. Which of the following is NOT associated with high hemoglobin concentrations (>13.2 g/dL)?

   a. preeclampsia in multiparas
   b. increased perinatal mortality
   c. increased low-birthweight infants
   d. increased preterm delivery

51–6. What are the most common causes of anemia during pregnancy?

   a. iron deficiency; acute blood loss
   b. iron deficiency; sickle cell disease
   c. folate deficiency; acute blood loss
   d. folate deficiency; sickle cell disease

51–7. Which of the following has the most influence on iron stores in the infant?

   a. maternal iron status
   b. timing of cord clamping
   c. maternal vitamin C intake
   d. blood loss at time of delivery

51–8. A peripheral smear in a black woman with a hemoglobin concentration of 8 g/dL reveals hypochromia and microcytosis. What is the most likely diagnosis?

   a. sickle cell anemia
   b. folate deficiency
   c. iron deficiency
   d. β-thalassemia

51–9. In the preceding patient, serum ferritin and iron-binding capacity are obtained. Which of the following confirms your diagnosis?

   a. low ferritin; decreased iron-binding capacity
   b. low ferritin; increased iron-binding capacity
   c. high ferritin; decreased iron-binding capacity
   d. high ferritin; increased iron-binding capacity

51–10. Which of the following excludes iron deficiency as a cause of anemia?

   a. elevated serum iron-binding capacity
   b. normal serum ferritin
   c. bone marrow normoblastic hyperplasia
   d. positive sickle cell prep

51–11. What is the treatment of iron-deficiency anemia during pregnancy?

    a. 50 mg elemental iron/day
    b. 100 mg elemental iron/day
    c. 200 mg elemental iron/day
    d. 400 mg elemental iron/day

51–12. What is the life span of the erythrocyte in anemias associated with chronic disease?

    a. does not change
    b. is longer by 20 to 30 days
    c. is longer by 50 to 70 days
    d. is shorter by 20 to 30 days

51–13. Which of the following is NOT associated with anemia?

    a. inflammatory bowel disease
    b. chronic renal disease
    c. essential hypertension
    d. systemic lupus erythematosus

51–14. In women with chronic renal disease, which of the following characterizes the degree of red cell mass expansion during pregnancy?

    a. is the same as in women with normal renal function
    b. is increased compared with normal pregnancy
    c. is decreased by the corresponding degree of renal impairment compared with normal pregnancy
    d. does not occur because of low levels of ferritin

51–15. What is the cause of anemia in women with acute antepartum pyelonephritis?

    a. decreased erythropoietin production
    b. increased red cell destruction due to endotoxemia
    c. dilution secondary to intravenous hydration
    d. decreased iron stores

51–16. What is the earliest morphological evidence of folic acid deficiency?

    a. hypersegmentation of neutrophils
    b. microcytosis

    c. macrocytic erythrocytes
    d. nucleated red blood cells

51–17. What is the treatment for pregnancy-induced megaloblastic anemia?

    a. nutritious diet only
    b. vitamin B_{12} 1000 μg every month
    c. iron (supplemental) 200 mg/day
    d. folic acid 1 mg/day, nutritious diet, and iron

51–18. In which of the following circumstances is supplemental folate not indicated?

    a. multifetal pregnancy
    b. Crohn's disease
    c. iron-deficiency anemia
    d. previous infant with neural-tube defect

51–19. Serum vitamin B_{12} levels are decreased in pregnancy secondary to which of the following?

    a. increased fibrinogen
    b. decreased fibrinogen
    c. increased transcobalamin
    d. decreased transcobalamin

51–20. What is the treatment for pregnant women who have undergone a total gastrectomy?

    a. 1 μg vitamin B_{12}
    b. 1000 μg vitamin B_{12}
    c. 1 mg folic acid
    d. 4 mg folic acid

51–21. What is the most common cause of autoimmune hemolytic anemia?

    a. drug-induced cold autoantibodies
    b. chronic inflammatory disease
    c. warm, active autoantibodies
    d. connective tissue disease

51–22. What is effective therapy for autoimmune hemolytic anemia?

    a. corticosteroids (e.g., prednisone 1 mg/kg/day)
    b. supplemental iron 200 mg/day
    c. folate 1 mg/day
    d. corticosteroids plus vitamin B_{12}

51–23. Which of the following is a hemopoietic stem-cell disorder characterized by formation of defective platelets, granulocytes, and erythrocytes?

    a. pregnancy-induced hemolytic anemia
    b. paroxysmal nocturnal hemoglobinuria
    c. autoimmune hemolytic anemia
    d. Diamond–Blackfan syndrome

51–24. On which of the following chromosomes is the abnormal gene for paroxysmal nocturnal hemoglobinuria located?

    a. 6
    b. 11
    c. 16
    d. X

51–25. What is the treatment of paroxysmal nocturnal hemoglobinuria?

    a. iron
    b. corticosteroids
    c. heparin
    d. bone marrow transplantation

51–26. What is the most common cause of aplastic anemia?

    a. drug-induced
    b. infection
    c. immunological disorder
    d. idiopathic effect

51–27. What is the major risk to a pregnant woman with aplastic anemia?

    a. infection
    b. preterm labor
    c. pregnancy-induced hypertension
    d. anemia

51–28. Which of the following is the therapy of choice for aplastic anemia if a suitable bone marrow donor is not available?

    a. corticosteroids
    b. testosterone
    c. antithymocyte globulin
    d. cytoxan

51–29. Hemoglobin S is owing to a substitution of which of the following?

    a. valine for glutamic acid at position 6
    b. glutamic acid for valine at position 6

    c. lysine for glutamic acid at position 6
    d. glutamic acid for leucine at position 6

51–30. What is the theoretical incidence of sickle cell anemia among African-Americans?

    a. 1 in 12
    b. 1 in 144
    c. 1 in 576
    d. 1 in 2000

51–31. Approximately how many African-Americans have the gene for hemoglobin C?

    a. 1 in 12
    b. 1 in 40
    c. 1 in 100
    d. 1 in 200

51–32. What is the approximate perinatal mortality in pregnancies complicated by sickle cell anemia and hemoglobin SC disease?

    a. 10 in 1000
    b. 100 in 1000
    c. 200 in 1000
    d. 500 in 1000

51–33. Which of the following is NOT associated with hemoglobin SC disease in pregnancy?

    a. severe bone pain
    b. pulmonary infarction
    c. placental abruption
    d. adult respiratory distress syndrome

51–34. Which of the following is NOT considered effective in the management of pain from intravascular sickling?

    a. intravenous hydration
    b. morphine
    c. prophylactic red cell transfusions
    d. therapeutic red cell transfusions

51–35. What is the chief benefit of prophylactic red cell transfusions in women with sickle cell anemia?

    a. decreased perinatal mortality
    b. decreased maternal morbidity
    c. decreased fetal growth retardation
    d. decreased preterm delivery

51–36. In patients with sickle cell disease, what is the incidence of isoimmunization per unit of blood transfused?

  a. 1%
  b. 3%
  c. 10%
  d. 30%

51–37. Which of the following is increased in pregnancies complicated by sickle cell trait?

  a. perinatal mortality
  b. abortion (spontaneous)
  c. low birthweight
  d. urinary tract infection

51–38. Which of the following adverse pregnancy outcomes is increased in women with hemoglobin C trait?

  a. preterm deliveries
  b. fetal growth retardation
  c. perinatal mortality
  d. not associated with adverse pregnancy outcome

51–39. Which of the following peripheral blood smears would be expected in a patient with hemoglobin E?

  a. hypochromia; microcytosis; erythrocyte targeting
  b. hypochromia; macrocytosis; erythrocyte targeting
  c. hypochromia; microcytosis; hypersegmented neutrophils
  d. hypochromia; macrocytosis; hypersegmented neutrophils

51–40. Which chromosome contains the gene for β-globin chain synthesis?

  a. 6
  b. 11
  c. 16
  d. 21

51–41. Which of the following characterizes thalassemias?

  a. impaired production of globin chains
  b. increased destruction of erythrocytes containing hemoglobin F
  c. increased production of globin chains
  d. decreased production of hemoglobin F

51–42. Which chromosome contains the gene for α-globin chain synthesis?

  a. 6
  b. 11
  c. 16
  d. 21

51–43. Which of the following patterns characterizes hemoglobin Bart?

  a. - -, a a
  b. - a, - a
  c. β4
  d. γ4

51–44. Which of the following ethnic groups is most likely to have hemoglobin Bart?

  a. Caucasians of Mediterranean descent
  b. Orientals
  c. Africans
  d. Greeks

51–45. What is the hallmark of β-thalassemias?

  a. elevated hemoglobin A
  b. elevated hemoglobin A_2
  c. elevated hemoglobin F
  d. elevated hemoglobin H

51–46. Which of the following characterizes β-thalassemia?

  a. increased β-chain production; decreased α chains
  b. increased β-chain production; increased α chains
  c. decreased β-chain production; decreased α chains
  d. decreased β-chain production; increased α chains

51–47. How is spherocytosis inherited?

  a. autosomal recessive
  b. autosomal dominant
  c. X-linked recessive
  d. X-linked dominant

51–48. How is glucose-6-phosphate dehydrogenase deficiency inherited?

  a. autosomal recessive
  b. autosomal dominant

c. X-linked recessive
d. X-linked dominant

51–49. Which of the following helps to differentiate polycythemia vera from secondary polycythemia?

    a. low values of erythropoietin in polycythemia vera (PCV)
    b. low values of erythropoietin in secondary polycythemia
    d. peripheral smear with nucleated erythropoietin
    d. peripheral smear with hypersegmented neutrophils in polycythemia vera

51–50. Which of the following causes of thrombocytopenia is owing to a lack of platelet membrane glycoprotein?

    a. May–Hegglin anomaly
    b. Bernand–Soulier syndrome
    c. hemolytic uremic syndrome
    d. drug-induced thrombocytopenia

51–51. What is the mechanism of action of gamma globulin in the therapy of immunological thrombocytopenia purpura?

    a. suppresses phagocytic activity in the spleen
    b. decreases removal of platelets by the spleen
    c. short-term reticuloendothelial blockade and diminishes platelet sequestration
    d. increases platelet production

51–52. What is the mechanism of action in corticosteroids for immune thrombocytopenia?

    a. stimulate platelet production
    b. block platelet antibodies
    c. suppress phagocytic activity
    d. unknown

51–53. What is the neonatal risk of maternal immune thrombocytopenia purpura?

    a. increased abortion rate
    b. thrombocytopenia
    c. necrotizing enterocolitis
    d. no risk

51–54. Which of the findings in women with immune thrombocytopenia purpura correlates absolutely with fetal platelet counts?

    a. maternal platelet count
    b. circulating antiplatelet antibodies
    c. indirect platelet antiglobulin
    d. no correlation with maternal status

51–55. What is the risk of neonatal thrombocytopenia in women with chronic immunological thrombocytopenia?

    a. 3%
    b. 10%
    c. 20%
    d. 30%

51–56. What is the average platelet count in women with essential thrombocytosis?

    a. 200,000
    b. 400,000
    c. 800,000
    d. 1,000,000

51–57. Which of the following is NOT a treatment for thrombocytosis complicating pregnancy?

    a. aspirin
    b. coumadin
    c. heparin
    d. dipyridamole

51–58. Which of the following is NOT part of the tetrad of thrombotic thrombocytopenic purpura?

    a. fever
    b. neurological abnormalities
    c. hemolytic anemia
    d. liver abnormalities

51–59. What is the pathogenesis of thrombotic microangiopathies?

    a. unknown
    b. microthrombi of hyaline material and platelets producing fluctuating ischemia
    c. microthrombi (multiple) of erythrocyte clumps causing multiple infarctions
    d. intravascular neutrophil aggregation stimulating cytokine production leading to end-organ failure

51–60. What is the most common presenting symptom in women with thrombotic thrombocytopenic syndrome?

a. fever
b. fatigue
c. hemorrhage
d. neurological abnormalities

51–61. What is the most common laboratory finding in women with thrombotic thrombocytopenic syndrome?

a. anemia
b. red cell fragmentation
c. leukocytes
d. fibrin-split products

51–62. What is the treatment for thrombotic thrombocytopenic syndromes?

a. heparin
b. aspirin and dipyridamole
c. glucocorticoids
d. exchange transfusion with donor plasma and plasmapheresis

51–63. What is the perinatal mortality in pregnancies complicated by thrombotic thrombocytopenic syndromes?

a. 20%
b. 40%
c. 60%
d. 80%

51–64. Which factor is deficient in individuals with hemophilia A?

a. von Willebrand factor
b. antithrombin III
c. factor VIII:C
d. factor IX

51–65. What is the most commonly inherited bleeding disorder?

a. von Willebrand disease
b. antithrombin III deficiency
c. factor VIII:C deficiency
d. factor IX deficiency

51–66. What is the site of synthesis of von Willebrand factor?

a. liver
b. endothelium and megakaryocytes
c. megakaryocytes only
d. kidney

51–67. How is protein C deficiency inherited?

a. X-linked recessive
b. autosomal recessive
c. autosomal dominant
d. multifactorial

51–68. What is the frequency of activated protein C resistance?

a. <0.1%
b. 0.5 to 1.0%
c. 3.0 to 7.0%
d. 10.0 to 12.0%

52

Diabetes

52–1. What year did insulin become available?

    a. 1906
    b. 1922
    c. 1932
    d. 1948

52–2. What is the concordance rates for type 1 diabetes in monozygotic twins?

    a. 100%
    b. 80%
    c. 60%
    d. <50%

52–3. Which of the following is the characteristic incidence of type 2 diabetes in monozygotic twins?

    a. 100%
    b. 80%
    c. 60%
    d. >50%

52–4. Which of the following is characteristic of type 2 diabetes?

    a. has absence of the islet cells
    b. shows destruction of the islet cells
    c. exhibits insulin resistance in target tissues
    d. develops ketoacidosis if untreated

52–5. Type 1 diabetes is associated with HLA-D histocompatibility complex located on which chromosome?

    a. 3
    b. 6
    c. 21
    d. 22

52–6. In general, what does glycosuria in pregnancy mean?

    a. represents lactose
    b. indicates diabetes
    c. usually is the result of a lowered renal threshold
    d. should be treated immediately with insulin

52–7. Which of the following is NOT a risk factor for gestational diabetes?

    a. age > 30 years
    b. prior macrosomic infant
    c. prior stillborn infant
    d. sister with gestational diabetes

52–8. According to the American College of Obstetricians and Gynecologists, screening for diabetes is recommended for all but which of the following?

    a. age > 30
    b. family history of diabetes
    c. prior macrosomia
    d. all pregnant women

52–9. What cutoff for the 50-g glucose screen would improve its sensitivity to 100 percent for detection of gestational diabetes?

    a. 130 mg/dL
    b. 135 mg/dL
    c. 140 mg/dL
    d. 145 mg/dL

52–10. What percentage of gestational diabetes will eventually develop into overt diabetes?

    a. none
    b. 10
    c. 25
    d. 50

52–11. In diabetes, which fetal organ is unaffected by fetal macrosomia?

    a. heart
    b. kidney
    c. liver
    d. brain

52–12. Which of the following is true concerning gestational diabetes?

    a. is increased with obesity
    b. has a prevalence of 1 to 3%
    c. with appropriate treatment has a normal perinatal mortality rate
    d. all of the above

52–13. How do you diagnose gestational diabetes?

    a. the 1 hour value of 50-g load of glucose exceeds 140 mg/dL
    b. elevated fasting value with a 100-g load of glucose
    c. elevated 1 hour value with a 100-g load of glucose
    d. two abnormal values are noted with a 100-g glucose tolerance test

52–14. What is the caloric requirement for a woman with gestational diabetes?

    a. 20 to 25 kcal/kg ideal body weight
    b. 30 to 35 kcal/kg ideal body weight
    c. 20 to 24 kcal/kg actual body weight
    d. 30 to 35 kcal/kg actual body weight

52–15. What are the benefits of postprandial glucose surveillance?

    a. better glucose control
    b. less neonatal hypoglycemia
    c. less macrosomia
    d. all of the above

52–16. What is the recurrence rate for gestational diabetes in subsequent pregnancies?

    a. 33%
    b. 50%
    c. 67%
    d. 90%

52–17. With the American College of Obstetricians and Gynecologists' classification of diabetes (1986), Class R includes which of the following?

    a. retinopathy
    b. proliferative retinopathy
    c. renal impairment
    d. onset before 10 years of age and duration for more than 20 years

52–18. With gestational diabetes, what is the most significant fetal consequence?

    a. congenital heart defects
    b. neural tube defects
    c. macrosomia
    d. chromosomal defects

52–19. When compared to normal pregnancy, which of the following is true concerning preeclampsia–eclampsia in a pregnancy with diabetes?

    a. less likely
    b. increased 2-fold
    c. increased 3-fold
    d. increased 4-fold

52–20. Which of the following is true concerning preconceptional glucose control in overt diabetic women?

    a. may reduce congenital anomalies
    b. may reduce spontaneous abortions
    c. still has a greater congenital anomaly rate than in nondiabetics
    d. all of the above

52–21. What is the most common birth defect in women with overt diabetes?

    a. chromosomal abnormality
    b. shortened cauda equina
    c. neural tube defects
    d. congenital heart defects

52–22. In general, when should overt diabetic pregnant women be delivered?

    a. 34 weeks
    b. 36 weeks
    c. 38 weeks
    d. 40 weeks

52–23. With which diabetic complication may pregnancy have a detrimental effect?

    a. proliferation retinopathy
    b. nephropathy
    c. hypertension
    d. nonproliferative retinopathy

52–24. What is the incidence of diabetic ketoacidosis during pregnancy?

    a. 0.5%
    b. 1.0%
    c. 3.0%
    d. 5.0%

52–25. How is overt diabetes diagnosed during pregnancy?

    a. 75-g GTT with two abnormal values
    b. 100-g GTT with two abnormal values
    c. fasting plasma glucose exceeding 95 on two occasions
    d. fasting plasma glucose exceeding 105 on two occasions

52–26. What is the most appropriate method of contraception for a diabetic patient?

    a. abstinence
    b. oral contraceptives
    c. intrauterine device
    d. sterilization

52–27. Which is true concerning terbutaline given to a gestational diabetic at 30 weeks?

    a. will increase the pulse rate
    b. will increase plasma glucose
    c. is not approved for tocolysis by the Food and Drug Administration
    d. all of the above

52–28. Which of the following is responsible for the diabetogenic effects of pregnancy?

    a. placental lactogen
    b. estrogens
    c. progesterone
    d. placental insulinase

52–29. Which of the following is least responsible for the diabetogenic effects of pregnancy?

    a. placental lactogen
    b. estrogen
    c. progesterone
    d. placental insulinase

53

Endocrine Disorders

53–1. What is the frequency of nontoxic goiter?

    a. 0.5%
    b. 2.0%
    c. 5.0%
    d. 10.0%

53–2. The thyroid undergoes which of the following changes during pregnancy?

    a. enlarges
    b. decreases in size
    c. remains the same size
    d. becomes nodular

53–3. Which of the following remains unchanged during pregnancy?

    a. total T_3 concentration
    b. total T_4 concentration
    c. serum thyrotropin
    d. thyroid-binding globulin

53–4. What is the role of chorionic thyrotropin in thyroid stimulation?

    a. marked stimulation
    b. slight stimulation
    c. no effect
    d. unclear

53–5. What is the incidence of thyrotoxicosis during pregnancy?

    a. 1 in 100
    b. 1 in 850
    c. 1 in 2000
    d. 1 in 10,000

53–6. Which of the following drugs has been reported to cause fetal hyperthyroidism and hypothyroidism?

    a. amiodarone
    b. propranolol
    c. captopril
    d. verapamil

53–7. What is the primary treatment for thyrotoxicosis during pregnancy?

    a. medical
    b. surgical
    c. combination of medical and surgical
    d. no treatment necessary

53–8. Which of the following medications causes *aplasia cutis*?

    a. propylthiouracil
    b. methimazole
    c. verapamil
    d. captopril

53–9. Following initiation of one of the thioamide drugs for hyperthyroidism, what is the median time to normalization of the free thyroxine index?

    a. 1 to 2 weeks
    b. 3 to 4 weeks
    c. 7 to 8 weeks
    d. 12 to 14 weeks

53–10. What is the reported perinatal mortality rate in women with thyrotoxicosis?

    a. 1 to 2%
    b. 8 to 12%

    c. 18 to 22%
    d. 25%

53–11. Which of the following drugs should be avoided in women with thyroid storm?

    a. acetaminophen
    b. salicylates
    c. propylthiouracil
    d. potassium iodide

53–12. Which of the following drugs may prove especially useful for the treatment of thyroid storm?

    a. propranolol
    b. esmolol
    c. methimazole
    d. verapamil

53–13. In one series of over 200 women treated with thiourea drugs, what was the incidence of adverse fetal effects?

    a. less than 2%
    b. 5 to 7%
    c. 12 to 15%
    d. 25%

53–14. In long-term studies of children born to thyrotoxic mothers treated with propylthiouracil during pregnancy, what was the finding regarding adverse effects?

    a. increase in adverse intellectual development
    b. increase in adverse physical development
    c. increase in adverse thyroid function
    d. no adverse effects

53–15. What percentage of women with gestational trophoblastic disease will have clinically apparent hyperthyroidism?

    a. 2%
    b. 8%
    c. 16%
    d. 25%

53–16. Which of the following complications is NOT increased in pregnant women with hypothyroidism?

    a. preeclampsia
    b. placental abruption

c. low birthweight

d. placenta previa

53–17. Women with which of the following medical complications have an increased risk of subclinical hypothyroidism?

a. chronic hypertension

b. renal disease

c. lupus erythematosus

d. type 1 diabetes

53–18. What is the risk of fetal anomalies in fetuses of mothers who have previously been treated (prior to pregnancy) with therapeutic radioiodine?

a. 6%

b. 8%

c. 12%

d. not increased

53–19. What percentage of states require biochemical screening of newborns for hypothyroidism?

a. 25%

b. 50%

c. 75%

d. 100%

53–20. What is the frequency of congenital hypothyroidism?

a. 1 in 40 to 70 infants

b. 1 in 400 to 700 infants

c. 1 in 4000 to 7000 infants

d. 1 in 40,000 to 70,000 infants

53–21. What percentage of thyroid nodules during pregnancy will be malignant?

a. 12%

b. 26%

c. 40%

d. 65%

53–22. What percentage of women will have either clinical or biochemical evidence of thyroid dysfunction during the postpartum period?

a. 1 to 2

b. 5 to 10

c. 18 to 20

d. 33

53–23. What percentage of women will have microsomal autoantibodies either early in pregnancy or shortly following delivery?

a. 1 to 2

b. 7 to 10

c. 19 to 20

d. 35

53–24. What is the role of calcitonin?

a. increases calcium

b. decreases calcium

c. keeps calcium at a steady level

d. has no effect on calcium

53–25. What happens to parathyroid hormone during pregnancy?

a. increases

b. decreases

c. stays the same

d. unclear

53–26. Which of the following is NOT a symptom of hypercalcemia?

a. fatigue

b. depression

c. diarrhea

d. nausea and vomiting

53–27. Which of the following is generally NOT utilized for the treatment of hypercalcemic crisis?

a. furosemide

b. mithramycin

c. oral phosphorus

d. propranolol

53–28. What is the primary treatment of hypoparathyroidism during pregnancy?

a. calcitriol

b. vitamin K

c. phosphorus

d. calcitonin

53–29. Which of the following hormones is probably NOT increased during pregnancy?

a. cortisol

b. renin

c. aldosterone

d. adrenal medullary hormone

53–30. What percentage of pheochromocytomas are bilateral, extraadrenal, and malignant?

    a. 1
    b. 10
    c. 20
    d. 40

53–31. Which of the following laboratory tests is NOT useful for the diagnosis of pheochromocytomas?

    a. cortisol
    b. vanillylmandelic acid
    c. metanephrine
    d. unconjugated catecholamines

53–32. Which of the following drugs is useful for the treatment of pheochromocytoma?

    a. α-methyl dopa
    b. phenoxybenzamine
    c. captopril
    d. verapamil

53–33. What is the most common cause of Addison's disease?

    a. tuberculosis
    b. histoplasmosis
    c. nonspecific granulomatous disease
    d. idiopathic autoimmune adrenalitis

53–34. What is the most common cause of Cushing syndrome in pregnancy?

    a. iatrogenic effect
    b. benign adrenal tumors
    c. adrenal carcinomas
    d. trophoblastic disease

53–35. Bromocriptine has proven efficacious for which of the following conditions during pregnancy?

    a. Graves' disease
    b. Addison's disease

    c. primary aldosteronism
    d. pituitary prolactinomas

53–36. What is the cutoff size used to distinguish a pituitary microadenoma from a macroadenoma?

    a. 5 mm
    b. 10 mm
    c. 50 mm
    d. 100 mm

53–37. What is the adverse fetal effect of bromocriptine?

    a. increase in stillbirths
    b. increase in growth retardation
    c. increase in microcephaly
    d. no adverse effect

53–38. What is the specific drug used to treat diabetes insipidus during pregnancy?

    a. DDAVP
    b. renin
    c. oxytocin
    d. angiotensin

53–39. Transient diabetes insipidus is most likely encountered in pregnant women with which of the following complications?

    a. acute fatty liver
    b. severe preeclampsia
    c. HELLP syndrome
    d. hemolytic uremic syndrome

53–40. Which of the following syndromes is caused by pituitary ischemia and necrosis secondary to obstetrical blood loss?

    a. Budd–Chiari syndrome
    b. Cushing syndrome
    c. Sheehan syndrome
    d. multiple endocrinopathy syndrome

54

Connective Tissue Disorders

54–1. Which of the following is an inherited non-inflammatory disorder of collagen metabolism?

    a. systemic lupus erythematosus (SLE)
    b. scleroderma
    c. Ehlers–Danlos syndrome
    d. rheumatoid arthritis

54–2. On which chromosome is the human leukocyte-associated (HLA) complex located?

    a. 6p
    b. 11p
    c. 14q
    d. 17q

54–3. Which of the following is a class II antigen?

    a. HLA-A
    b. HLA-B
    c. HLA-C
    d. HLA-DR

54–4. What happens to serum levels of autoantibodies during pregnancy?

    a. increase
    b. decrease
    c. remain the same
    d. unknown

54–5. What percentage of systemic lupus erythematosus occurs in women?

    a. 30
    b. 50
    c. 70
    d. 90

54–6. What is the frequency of lupus in women with one affected family member?

    a. 1%
    b. 2 to 3%
    c. 10%
    d. 25%

54–7. How many of the 11 criteria of the American Rheumatism Association must be present to make the diagnosis of lupus?

    a. 2
    b. 4
    c. 8
    d. 10

54–8. How many women with lupus have renal involvement?

    a. 10%
    b. 25%
    c. 50%
    d. 75%

54–9. What is the overall 10-year survival for women with lupus?

    a. 50%
    b. 65%
    c. 75%
    d. 90%

54–10. Which of the following is a common clinical manifestation of lupus?

    a. arthralgias
    b. seizures
    c. pleuritis
    d. venous thrombosis

54–11. Which is the best screening test for lupus?

    a. anti-SM antibodies
    b. cardiolipin antibodies
    c. antiplatelet antibodies
    d. antinuclear antibodies

54–12. Which of the following autoantibodies is specific for lupus?

    a. anti-RNA
    b. antinuclear
    c. anti-ds DNA
    d. anti-RNP

54–13. Which of the following is NOT a common laboratory finding in women with lupus?

    a. anemia
    b. positive indirect Coombs test
    c. hemolysis
    d. false-positive syphilis serology

54–14. Which of the following is the usual first-line therapy for lupus?

    a. steroids
    b. nonsteroidal anti-inflammatory drugs
    c. azathioprine
    d. cyclophosphamide

54–15. What is the most common complication in pregnant women with lupus nephritis?

    a. renal failure
    b. hypertension
    c. abruption
    d. fetal demise

54–16. In the management of lupus, azathioprine should be used in the presence of which of the following?

    a. seizures
    b. steroid-resistant nephropathy
    c. lupus activation
    d. thrombocytopenia

54–17. What is the incidence of newborn lupus caused by transplacental passage of IgG anti-SSA(Ro) and anti-SSB(La) antibodies?

    a. 10%
    b. 25%
    c. 50%
    d. rare

54–18. Which of the following maternal antibodies is/are associated with congenital heart block in the newborn?

    a. anti-SSA(Ro) and anti-SSB(La)
    b. anti-ds DNA

    c. ANA
    d. anti-RNA

54–19. What percentage of infants with congenital heart block secondary to lupus will die within the first 3 years of life?

    a. 5
    b. 15
    c. 33
    d. 50

54–20. Antibodies of which class are antiphospholipid antibodies?

    a. IgG
    b. IgM
    c. IgA
    d. all three

54–21. Approximately what percentage of women with lupus will have the lupus anticoagulant?

    a. 5
    b. 25
    c. 33
    d. 75

54–22. What percentage of women with anticardiolipin antibodies will have the lupus anticoagulant?

    a. 5
    b. 20
    c. 50
    d. 90

54–23. What percentage of normal pregnant women will have nonspecific antiphospholipid antibodies in low titers?

    a. <1
    b. 3 to 6
    c. 15
    d. 25

54–24. What is the most commonly used test for identifying antiphospholipid antibodies?

    a. PCR
    b. prothrombin time test
    c. ELISA
    d. monoclonal antibody test

54–25. Which clotting test is most specific for identifying the lupus anticoagulant?

   a. platelet neutralization procedure
   b. bleeding time test
   c. prothrombin time test
   d. partial thromboplastin time test

54–26. Which of the following is NOT associated with the lupus anticoagulant and antiphospholipid antibodies?

   a. venous thrombosis
   b. arterial thrombosis
   c. hemolytic anemia
   d. thrombocytosis

54–27. Which of the following treatment protocols appears to result in the best pregnancy outcome for women with the lupus anticoagulant?

   a. corticosteroids plus low-dose aspirin
   b. corticosteroids plus heparin
   c. heparin plus low-dose aspirin
   d. aspirin alone

54–28. What is the recommended treatment for pregnant women with antiphospholipid antibodies and a history of arterial thrombosis?

   a. low-dose heparin and low-dose aspirin
   b. low-dose aspirin only
   c. low-dose heparin only
   d. therapeutic anticoagulation

54–29. Which of the following HLA-haplotypes is associated with rheumatoid arthritis?

   a. HLA-DQ
   b. HLA-DR4
   c. HLA-DP
   d. HLA-DR2

54–30. What is the cornerstone of therapy for rheumatoid arthritis?

   a. aspirin
   b. corticosteroids
   c. sulfasalazine
   d. cyclosporine

54–31. What is the usual course of rheumatoid arthritis in pregnancy?

   a. not changed from baseline
   b. marked by gradual deterioration

   c. characterized by rapid deterioration
   d. characterized by marked improvement

54–32. Which of the following proteins/hormones may be responsible for the improvement in rheumatoid arthritis during pregnancy?

   a. cortisol
   b. estrogens
   c. pregnancy-associated α_2-glycoprotein
   d. human placental lactogen

54–33. What adverse perinatal outcome is associated with rheumatoid arthritis?

   a. stillbirth
   b. fetal growth retardation
   c. preterm birth
   d. none of the above

54–34. What is the hallmark of systemic sclerosis?

   a. increased production of fibrin
   b. increased production of collagen
   c. decreased macrophage activity
   d. increased autoantibody production

54–35. What percentage of women with scleroderma will have antinuclear antibodies?

   a. 5
   b. 20
   c. 50
   d. 90

54–36. What percentage of deaths associated with scleroderma are secondary to renal failure?

   a. 5
   b. 20
   c. 50
   d. 90

54–37. What is the treatment for systemic sclerosis?

   a. aspirin
   b. cortisol
   c. sulfasalazine
   d. no effective treatment

54–38. Which of the following vasculitis syndromes is associated with hepatitis B antigenemia?

   a. polyarthritis nodosa
   b. Wegener granulomatosis
   c. Grant-cell arteritis
   d. dermatomyositis

54–39. Which of the following syndromes is inherited by an autosomal dominant gene?

a. polymyositis
b. polyarteritis nodosa
c. Marfan syndrome
d. dermatomyositis

54–40. What percentage of adults developing dermatomyositis will have an associated malignant tumor?

a. 1 to 2
b. 15
c. 33
d. 50

54–41. Which of the following is characterized by hyperelasticity of the skin?

a. dermatomyositis
b. polyarteritis nodosa
c. Marfan syndrome
d. Ehlers-Danlos syndrome

54–42. Which of the following complications is increased in Ehlers-Danlos syndrome?

a. preterm ruptured fetal membranes
b. hypertension
c. eclampsia
d. twinning

55

Neurological and Psychiatric Disorders

55–1. What is the frequency of cerebral palsy in children of mothers with epilepsy compared to the general population?

a. increased
b. decreased
c. unchanged
d. unknown

55–2. What is the frequency of congenital malformations in children of mothers with epilepsy compared to the general population?

a. increased
b. decreased
c. unchanged
d. unknown

55–3. Which of the following anticonvulsants is most likely to be associated with a neural tube defect?

a. phenobarbital
b. carbamazepine
c. phenytoin
d. valproic acid

55–4. How should the dosage of phenytoin (Dilantin) generally be managed during pregnancy?

a. increased
b. decreased
c. not changed
d. monitored routinely with serum levels

55–5. Which of the following may be decreased in women with children who have the anticonvulsant embryopathy?

    a. vitamin A
    b. epoxide hydrolase
    c. serum calcium
    d. folic acid

55–6. Which of the following vitamins may be of benefit in preventing neonatal complications in newborns of mothers taking phenytoin?

    a. vitamin A
    b. vitamin D
    c. vitamin E
    d. vitamin K

55–7. What percentage of direct maternal deaths are caused by stroke?

    a. 1
    b. 10
    c. 18
    d. 29

55–8. What percentage of ischemic strokes are caused by antiphospholipid antibodies?

    a. 5
    b. 10
    c. 33
    d. 55

55–9. Which of the following conditions may be associated with sagittal venous sinus thrombosis?

    a. antithrombin III deficiency
    b. protein C deficiency
    c. protein S deficiency
    d. all of the above

55–10. When is venous thrombosis of the cerebral circulation most common?

    a. first trimester
    b. second trimester
    c. labor
    d. the puerperium

55–11. What is the most common source of cerebral artery embolism in pregnancy?

    a. femor artery
    b. uterine artery
    c. ovarian artery
    d. heart

55–12. What is the most common cause of subarachnoid hemorrhage during pregnancy?

    a. circulating anticoagulant
    b. chronic hypertension
    c. preeclampsia
    d. rupture of cerebral aneurysm or AVM

55–13. Bleeding from a ruptured aneurysm is most common during what part of pregnancy?

    a. first half
    b. second half
    c. labor
    d. puerperium

55–14. What percentage of unresected arteriovenous malformations will bleed again within the first year?

    a. 5
    b. 15
    c. 28
    d. 50

55–15. What is the usual course of migraine headaches during pregnancy?

    a. minimal improvement
    b. dramatic improvement
    c. minimal worsening
    d. dramatic worsening

55–16. Which of the following drugs should NOT be utilized for the treatment of migraine headaches during pregnancy?

    a. sumatriptan
    b. propranolol
    c. ergonovine
    d. amitriptyline

55–17. What percentage of women with multiple sclerosis will have an exacerbation during the first few months postpartum?

    a. 5
    b. 33
    c. 50
    d. 90

55–18. How is Huntington's disease inherited?

   a. autosomal dominant
   b. autosomal recessive
   c. X-linked recessive
   d. multifactorial

55–19. Which of the following drugs is used in the treatment of myasthenia gravis?

   a. pyridostigmine
   b. propranolol
   c. indomethacin
   d. nifedipine

55–20. Women with myasthenia gravis frequently have hyperplasia of which of the following organs?

   a. liver
   b. thymus
   c. adrenal
   d. pituitary

55–21. Which of the following antibiotics should be utilized with caution in pregnant women with myasthenia gravis?

   a. penicillin
   b. cefalosporins
   c. aminoglycosides
   d. sulfonamides

55–22. What percentage of newborns will develop neonatal myasthenia gravis?

   a. 2
   b. 15
   c. 33
   d. 65

55–23. What percentage of Guillain-Barré syndrome results from a viral infection?

   a. 10
   b. 33
   c. 66
   d. 90

55–24. What percentage of women with Guillain-Barré syndrome will have full recovery?

   a. 50
   b. 66
   c. 85
   d. 99

55–25. What percentage of women with hand symptoms actually have evidence of median nerve compression (i.e., carpal tunnel syndrome)?

   a. 5
   b. 20
   c. 50
   d. 70

55–26. Which of the following is NOT a complication of spinal cord injury?

   a. anemia
   b. urinary infection
   c. pressure necrosis of the skin
   d. diarrhea

55–27. Autonomic hyperreflexia is generally associated with a spinal cord injury above what level?

   a. T_5-T_6
   b. T_7
   c. T_{10}
   d. T_{12}

55–28. Which of the following is NOT associated with autonomic hyperreflexia?

   a. headache
   b. facial flushing
   c. hypertension
   d. bradycardia

55–29. Which of the following is utilized to decrease the frequency of autonomic hyperreflexia?

   a. nifedipine
   b. propranolol
   c. general anesthesia
   d. epidural/spinal

55–30. Which of the following is NOT a sign or symptom of pseudotumor cerebri?

   a. deafness
   b. visual disturbances
   c. papilledema
   d. stiff neck

55–31. Which of the following drugs is utilized for the treatment of pseudotumor cerebri?

   a. propranolol
   b. acetazolamide

c. captopril
d. nifedipine

55–32. What percentage of women will have a nonpsychotic postpartum depressive disorder?

    a. 10 to 15
    b. 20 to 25
    c. 45 to 50
    d. 65 to 70

55–33. What type of disorder is manic–depressive illness?

    a. emotional
    b. personality
    c. unipolar
    d. bipolar

55–34. If one parent is schizophrenic, what is the empirical risk to their offspring of such a disorder?

    a. 1 to 2%
    b. 5 to 10%
    c. 65%
    d. 89%

55–35. What percentage of pregnant women will experience postpartum blues?

    a. 5
    b. 15
    c. 30
    d. 50

55–36. What is the recurrence risk of postpartum depression?

    a. 5%
    b. 20%
    c. 70%
    d. 95%

55–37. What is the recurrence risk of postpartum psychosis?

    a. 5%
    b. 25%
    c. 50%
    d. 75%

55–38. Which of the following psychotropic medications may be associated with Ebstein anomaly?

    a. amitriptyline
    b. impramine
    c. chlorpromazine
    d. lithium

56

Dermatological Disorders

56–1. Hyperpigmentation of pregnancy is related to which of the following?

    a. cortisol
    b. aldosterone
    c. melanocyte-stimulating hormone
    d. unknown

56–2. Which of the following best describes telogen effluvium?

    a. caused by high levels of melanocyte-stimulating hormone
    b. self-limiting and resolved in 6 to 12 months
    c. associated with oral contraceptives
    d. all of the above

56–3. What is chloasma?

    a. pigmentation of the areolae
    b. pigmentation of the linea alba
    c. pigmentation of the face
    d. pigmentation of the inner thigh

56–4. Which of the following hormones most likely causes spider angiomas during pregnancy?

    a. estrogen
    b. progesterone
    c. cortisol
    d. chorionic gonadotropin

56–5. Which of the following conditions results from a mild form of cholestatic jaundice?

    a. pruritis gravidarum
    b. capillary hemangiomas
    c. palmar erythema
    d. pruritic urticarial papules and plaques of pregnancy (PUPPP)

56–6. What is the usual treatment for PUPPP?

    a. corticosteroids
    b. benzoyl peroxide
    c. zinc oxide
    d. topical tretinoin

56–7. Herpes gestationis may be associated with which of the following?

    a. chorioangioma
    b. trophoblastic disease
    c. preeclampsia
    d. herpes zoster

56–8. What is the effect of herpes gestationis on fetal outcome?

    a. increased
    b. decreased if on steroids
    c. no effect
    d. unclear

56–9. Of the following, which is most likely associated with Graves' disease?

    a. pruritus gravidarum
    b. pruritic urticarial papules and plaques of pregnancy
    c. herpes gestationis
    d. impetigo herpetiformis

56–10. Which of the following is a form of pustular psoriasis?

    a. pruritis gravidarum
    b. herpes gestationis
    c. impetigo herpetiformis
    d. psoriasis gravidarum

56–11. The spongioform pustule of Kogoj is most likely caused by which of the following?

    a. *Staphylococcus aureus*
    b. β-*Streptococcus*
    c. *E. coli*
    d. none of the above

56–12. Which of the following is an FDA category B drug?

    a. isotretinoin
    b. etretinate
    c. topical tretinoin
    d. benzoyl peroxide

57

Neoplastic Diseases

57–1. What is the approximate incidence of cancer in pregnancy?

    a. 1 in 500
    b. 1 in 5000
    c. 1 in 50,000
    d. 1 in 500,000

57–2. What is the earliest gestational age at which the ovaries may be removed safely because placental progesterone production is adequate?

    a. 4 weeks
    b. 6 weeks
    c. 8 weeks
    d. 12 weeks

57–3. What is the characteristic adverse effect of high-dose radiation in pregnancy?

    a. leukemia
    b. radiation nephritis
    c. microcephaly and mental retardation
    d. fetal cardiac defects

57–4. Negligible risk from radiation for major malformations is noted as below which of the following doses?

    a. 5 rad
    b. 10 rad
    c. 15 rad
    d. 20 rad

57–5. Antineoplastic drugs are most hazardous when given at what gestational age?

    a. first trimester
    b. second trimester
    c. just before delivery
    d. postpartum breast feeding

57–6. What is the major risk from multidrug regimens for Hodgkin lymphoma?

    a. ovarian fibrosis
    b. abortion
    c. fetal chromosomal damage
    d. fetal anomalies

57–7. How common is breast cancer during pregnancy?

    a. most common cancer
    b. second most common cancer
    c. fourth most common cancer
    d. rare cause of cancer during pregnancy

57–8. Stage for stage, what influence does pregnancy have on the course of breast cancer?

    a. decreases survival
    b. increases survival
    c. no influence
    d. unknown

57–9. What is the incidence of lymphoma in a woman with human immunodeficiency virus (HIV)?

    a. same as in the general population
    b. 1%
    c. 5 to 10%
    d. 15 to 20%

57–10. Approximately what percentage of pregnant women with breast cancer will have nodal involvement?

    a. 25
    b. 50
    c. 75
    d. 90

57–11. What is the radiation exposure to the fetus from mammography?

    a. <1 rad
    b. 5 rad
    c. 10 rad
    d. 25 rad

57–12. Which of the following is NOT a recommended therapy for breast cancer during pregnancy?

    a. mastectomy
    b. mastectomy and node dissection
    c. chemotherapy
    d. radiotherapy

57–13. What is the recommended delay for future pregnancy following treatment of breast cancer?

    a. 6 months to one year
    b. 2 to 3 years
    c. 5 years
    d. 7 to 8 years

57–14. Pregnant women with Hodgkin disease are inordinately susceptible to which of the following complications?

    a. infection
    b. renal failure
    c. breast cancer
    d. ovarian cancer

57–15. Approximately what percentage of women treated for Hodgkin disease with chemotherapy will resume normal menses?

    a. 10
    b. 20
    c. 50
    d. 90

57–16. What percentage of women with Hodgkin disease will develop leukemia within 15 years?

    a. 5
    b. 20
    c. 39
    d. 55

57–17. What is the incidence of leukemia in pregnancy?

    a. 1 per 1000
    b. 1 per 10,000

    c. 1 per 100,000
    d. 1 per 1,000,000

57–18. What percentage of pregnant women with acute leukemia will have a remission with chemotherapy?

    a. 10
    b. 25
    c. 40
    d. 75

57–19. How long should pregnancy be avoided following treatment for melanoma?

    a. 1 to 2 years
    b. 3 to 5 years
    c. 8 to 10 years
    d. should not become pregnant

57–20. What is the most common form of cancer encountered during pregnancy?

    a. breast
    b. melanoma
    c. hematologic
    d. genital

57–21. What is the diagnostic accuracy of colposcopically directed biopsy during pregnancy?

    a. 20%
    b. 66%
    c. 84%
    d. 99%

57–22. How does pregnancy affect the survival rate for invasive carcinoma of the cervix?

    a. increases
    b. decreases
    c. no effect
    d. unknown

57–23. What effect does vaginal delivery through a cancerous cervix have on the prognosis?

    a. better than with cesarean delivery
    b. worse than with cesarean delivery
    c. no different than with cesarean delivery
    d. unknown

57–24. What percentage of adnexal neoplasms during pregnancy are malignant?

    a. <1
    b. 5

c. 20

d. 38

57–25. Which is the most common ovarian neoplasm associated with pregnancy?

a. epithelial

b. germ cell

c. stromal

d. miscellaneous

57–26. What percentage of colon cancers are palpable by rectal examination?

a. 20 to 25

b. 25 to 40

c. 60 to 70

d. 88 to 95

$\boxed{58}$

Infections

58–1. At what stage of gestation does fetal humoral immunity begin to develop?

a. 4 to 8 weeks

b. 9 to 15 weeks

c. 17 to 24 weeks

d. 36 to 40 weeks

58–2. What percentage of pregnant women with primary varicella infection develop pneumonitis?

a. <1

b. 10

c. 25

d. 40

58–3. In varicella-exposed susceptible immunocompromised individuals, the Centers for Disease Control and Prevention recommends prophylaxis with which of the following?

a. varicella vaccine

b. varicella-zoster immunoglobulin

c. immunoglobulin

d. gamma globulin

58–4. Which of the following is NOT part of the varicella embryopathy?

a. chorioretinitis

b. multicystic kidneys

c. limb atrophy

d. cortical atrophy

58–5. When should varicella zoster immunoglobulin be administered to the newborn?

a. if delivery is within 21 days of maternal disease

b. if delivery is within 10 days of maternal disease

c. if delivery is within 5 days of maternal disease

d. if maternal disease occurs at 7 days of newborn age

58–6. Which of the following agents has specific activity against influenza A?

a. amantadine

b. acyclovir

c. ganciclovir

d. adenosine araboside

58–7. Which of the following infections is owing to an RNA paramyxovirus?

   a. herpes
   b. mumps
   c. influenza
   d. varicella

58–8. What associated pregnancy complications are increased in women with measles?

   a. stillbirths
   b. abortions
   c. fetal anomalies
   d. abruptio placentas

58–9. Which of the following is likely to produce a cough and lower respiratory infection (i.e., pneumonia)?

   a. rhinovirus
   b. coronavirus
   c. echovirus
   d. adenovirus

58–10. What is the case fatality rate from the hantavirus?

   a. <10%
   b. 10%
   c. 35%
   d. 60%

58–11. Which of the following is NOT associated with Coxsackievirus viremia in the fetus?

   a. pancreatitis
   b. hepatitis
   c. myocarditis
   d. encephalomyelitis

58–12. Which of the following tests is used to confirm the diagnosis of erythema infectiosum?

   a. antistreptolysis titer
   b. parvovirus IgM titer
   c. rubella IgM titer
   d. coxsackievirus IgM

58–13. In which of the following situations might parvovirus be associated with aplastic crisis?

   a. iron-deficiency anemia
   b. thalassemia minor

   c. Gaucher disease
   d. sickle cell anemia

58–14. Which of the following adverse fetal effects has been reported to be caused by maternal parvovirus infection?

   a. microcephaly
   b. hydrocephaly
   c. hydrops
   d. cardiac defects

58–15. By how many days does rubella viremia precede clinically evident disease?

   a. 1 day
   b. 4 days
   c. 7 days
   d. 21 days

58–16. How long does rubella IgM persist?

   a. 14 days
   b. 28 days
   c. 60 days
   d. 90 days

58–17. Congenital rubella syndrome is more common during which weeks of gestation?

   a. 8 to 10 weeks
   b. 12 to 14 weeks
   c. 16 to 18 weeks
   d. 36 to 38 weeks

58–18. Which of the following is NOT part of the congenital rubella syndrome?

   a. cataracts
   b. septal defects
   c. sensorineural deafness
   d. pancreatitis

58–19. Which of the following is a handicap associated with cytomegalovirus infection?

   a. deafness
   b. diabetes
   c. cataracts
   d. spastic paralysis

58–20. What is the risk of cytomegalovirus seroconversion among susceptible women during pregnancy?

   a. <1%
   b. 1 to 4%

c. 10%
d. 20%

58–21. What is the rate of transmission to the fetus during primary cytomegalovirus infection?

a. 10%
b. 20%
c. 30%
d. 40%

58–22. Which of the following is NOT associated with cytomegalic inclusion disease?

a. microcephaly
b. chorioretinitis
c. hydrops
d. thrombocytopenic purpura

58–23. Which of the following is the most sensitive method to diagnose maternal primary CMV infection?

a. culture of cervix
b. cytomegalovirus IgG titer
c. cytomegalovirus IgM titer
d. 2-fold increase in IgG titer

58–24. Which of the following techniques is best to diagnose fetal CMV infection?

a. amniocentesis
b. chorionic villus sampling
c. sonography
d. magnetic resonance imaging

58–25. Which of the following is associated with *Streptococcus pyogenes* (group A streptococcus)?

a. toxic shocklike syndrome
b. scarlet fever
c. erysipelas
d. all of the above

58–26. What percentage of pregnant women are colonized with *Streptococcus agalactiae* (group B streptococcus [GBS])?

a. <1
b. 5 to 10
c. 15 to 20
d. 40 to 50

58–27. What is the attack rate for group B streptococcus in preterm babies born to colonized mothers?

a. 1 to 2 per 1000 live births
b. 10 per 1000 live births
c. 20 per 1000 live births
d. 40 per 1000 live births

58–28. Which of the following is NOT a characteristic of early onset group B streptococcus neonatal infection?

a. onset at 1 to 2 weeks of age
b. respiratory distress
c. apnea
d. shock

58–29. What is the most accurate method for detection of group B streptococcal infection?

a. Gram stain
b. latex agglutination test
c. culture
d. enzyme-linked immunosorbent assay

58–30. Which of the following are gram-positive aerobic bacilli?

a. *Streptococcus pyogenes*
b. *Listeria monocytogenes*
c. *Salmonella typhi*
d. *Streptococcus faecalis*

58–31. Which of the following is associated with fetal listeria infection?

a. osteochondritis
b. neuronal destruction
c. granulomatous lesions with microabscesses
d. myocarditis

58–32. What is the treatment of choice for listeria during the third trimester?

a. metronidazole
b. ampicillin plus gentamicin
c. clindamycin
d. tetracycline

58–33. Which of the following is generally used as the treatment for salmonella enteritis?

a. intravenous fluids
b. ampicillin
c. ampicillin plus gentamicin
d. ampicillin plus sulbactam

58–34. What is the attack rate for shigellosis?

    a. 10%
    b. 20%
    c. 40%
    d. 75%

58–35. What is the causative organism of Hansen disease?

    a. *Shigella hanseni*
    b. *Borrelia burgdorferi*
    c. *Mycobacterium leprae*
    d. *Toxoplasmosis gondii*

58–36. What is the causative organism for Lyme disease?

    a. *Treponoma pallidum*
    b. *Borrelia burgdorferi*
    c. *Borrelia ixodes*
    d. *Toxoplasma gondii*

58–37. What is the treatment of choice for Lyme disease in pregnancy?

    a. amoxicillin
    b. clindamycin
    c. gentamicin
    d. tetracycline

58–38. Which of the following organisms is associated with eating undercooked meat?

    a. *Borrelia burgdorferi*
    b. *Plasmodium vivax*
    c. *Mycobacterium leprae*
    d. *Toxoplasmosis gondii*

58–39. What is the overall risk of fetal infection from primary maternal toxoplasmosis?

    a. 5%
    b. 15%
    c. 50%
    d. 80%

58–40. What percentage of fetuses infected in the first trimester will have congenital toxoplasmosis?

    a. 3
    b. 10
    c. 40
    d. 70

58–41. Which of the following is associated with congenital toxoplasmosis infection?

    a. limb defects
    b. cardiac defects
    c. hepatosplenomegaly
    d. renal defects

58–42. How long can toxoplasmosis IgM persist?

    a. days
    b. weeks
    c. months
    d. years

58–43. Which of the following is potential treatment for toxoplasmosis in pregnancy?

    a. spectinomycin
    b. erythromycin
    c. sulfasalazine
    d. spiramycin

58–44. What is the treatment of choice for chloroquine-resistant falciparum infection?

    a. high-dose chloroquine
    b. chloramphenicol
    c. quinine
    d. mefloquine

59

Sexually Transmitted Diseases

59–1. Which of the following is true concerning syphilis in reproductive-age women?

    a. Rates peaked in 1950.
    b. Rates peaked in 1975.
    c. Rates peaked in 1990.
    d. Rates continue to rise.

59–2. Antepartum syphilis is NOT associated with which of the following?

    a. fetal death
    b. preterm labor
    c. neonatal infection
    d. abruptio placenta

59–3. What is the incubation period for primary syphilis?

    a. 1 day
    b. 1 week
    c. 10 to 90 days
    d. 6 months

59–4. Which of the following best describes the primary chancre?

    a. painless firm ulcer
    b. painful firm ulcer
    c. painless erythematous lesion
    d. painful erythematous lesion

59–5. What is the approximate time for development of secondary syphilis following healing of the primary chancre?

    a. 7 days
    b. 10 to 14 days
    c. 6 to 8 weeks
    d. 12 weeks or more

59–6. What is the characteristic lesion of secondary syphilis?

    a. condyloma lata
    b. multiple chancres

    c. massive vulvar ulcers
    d. none

59–7. At what gestational age does the fetus first manifest clinical disease if infected by syphilis?

    a. 6 weeks
    b. 8 to 10 weeks
    c. 12 weeks
    d. 18 weeks or more

59–8. What are syphilitic changes in the liver termed?

    a. condyloma hepaticum
    b. syphilitic hepatitis
    c. portal syphilis
    d. hypertrophic cirrhosis

59–9. After contracting the disease, when will serological tests for syphilis be positive?

    a. <7 days
    b. 10 to 14 days
    c. 28 to 42 days
    d. ~90 days

59–10. Which of the following is the most specific test for syphilis?

    a. fluorescent treponemal antibody absorption test (FTA-ABS)
    b. venereal disease research laboratory test (VDRL)
    c. rapid plasma reagin test (RPR)
    d. culture in rat ovaries

59–11. What is the best test for diagnosis of neonatal syphilis?

    a. cord blood VDRL
    b. motile spirochetes in amnionic fluid
    c. neonatal serum polymerase chain reaction
    d. sonographic evidence of large placenta

59–12. What is the treatment of choice for syphilis in pregnancy?

   a. tetracycline
   b. doxycycline
   c. erythromycin
   d. penicillin

59–13. Penicillin G cures what percentage of maternal infections and prevents what percentage of neonatal disease?

   a. 70
   b. 80
   c. 90
   d. 98

59–14. Syphilis of more than 1 year's duration should be treated with which of the following?

   a. penicillin V 250 mg po qid × 10 days
   b. benzathine penicillin G 2.4 million units IM
   c. benzathine penicillin G 2.4 million units IM weekly × 3
   d. aqueous penicillin G 4 million units every 4 hours for 10 days

59–15. What is the best alternative therapy for the treatment of syphilis in pregnant women who are allergic to penicillin?

   a. ceftriaxone
   b. erythromycin
   c. tetracycline
   d. penicillin desensitization

59–16. Which of the following antibiotics may be curative of syphilis in the mother but may not prevent congenital syphilis?

   a. penicillin
   b. erythromycin
   c. tetracycline
   d. ceftriaxone

59–17. Despite recommended treatment during pregnancy, what percentage of newborns of mothers with syphilis have obvious clinical stigmata of congenital syphilis?

   a. 2
   b. 5

   c. 20
   d. 44

59–18. How is the Jarisch–Herxheimer reaction in pregnancy characterized?

   a. hypotension
   b. uterine quiescence
   c. late fetal heart rate decelerations
   d. hypothermia

59–19. What is the best option for hydropic fetuses with congenital syphilis?

   a. Treat maternal infection.
   b. Administer early delivery and neonatal treatment.
   c. Wait for labor and treat intrapartum.
   d. Wait for delivery and reassess infant status.

59–20. In pregnant women with latent syphilis of more than 1 year's duration, which of the following is NOT one of the criteria for recommending lumbar puncture?

   a. neurological symptoms
   b. treatment failures
   c. concomitant HIV infection
   d. serological titer of 1 to 4

59–21. Which of the following treatment protocols is appropriate for the asymptomatic infant whose mother was treated with erythromycin for syphilis ?

   a. penicillin G, 50,000 U per kg × 10 days
   b. erythromycin 500 mg for 4 doses
   c. treatment only if symptoms are present
   d. no treatment necessary

59–22. Which of the following is a risk factor for gonorrhea?

   a. married
   b. age > 35
   c. multiparous
   d. lack of prenatal care

59–23. What percentage of pregnant women with gonorrhea will also have chlamydia?

   a. <5
   b. 20
   c. 40
   d. 60

59–24. Which of the following is NOT found with a higher prevalence in pregnant women with gonorrhea?

a. oropharyngeal infection
b. anal infection
c. tubo-ovarian abscess
d. disseminated infection

59–25. Which of the following is NOT associated with *Neisseria gonorrhoeae?*

a. preterm labor
b. chorioamnionitis
c. endometritis
d. abruptio placenta

59–26. What is the treatment of choice for uncomplicated gonorrhea in pregnancy?

a. ceftriaxone
b. penicillin
c. erythromycin
d. azithromycin

59–27. Which of the following is NOT a symptom or sign of disseminated gonococcal infection?

a. clear vesicular lesions
b. arthralgias
c. septic arthritis
d. tenosynovitis

59–28. Which of the following is an obligate intracellular bacterium?

a. *Treponema pallidum*
b. *Borrelia burgdorferi*
c. *Chlamydia trachomatis*
d. *Escherichia coli*

59–29. Which of the following is the most common sexually transmitted disease in women?

a. *Neisseria gonorrhoeae*
b. herpes
c. chancroid
d. *Chlamydia trachomatis*

59–30. What is the sensitivity of polymerase chain reaction for the detection of chlamydia?

a. 2%
b. 50%
c. 75%
d. 95%

59–31. What is NOT considered a risk factor for chlamydia infection?

a. age > 20
b. unmarried
c. lower socioeconomic group
d. multiple sex partners

59–32. Vertical transmission of chlamydia is associated with which of the following neonatal infections?

a. sepsis
b. conjunctivitis
c. urine infection
d. skin rash

59–33. In pregnancies complicated by chlamydia, which of the following is positively associated with poor pregnancy prognosis?

a. untreated cervical chlamydia
b. recent infection as evidenced by elevated IgM
c. history of treatment failure
d. all of the above

59–34. Which of the following organisms is associated with late-onset postpartum endometritis?

a. *Neisseria gonorrhoeae*
b. *Fusobacterium* sp.
c. *Mycoplasma* sp.
d. *Chlamydia trachomatis*

59–35. What percentage of infants born through an infected cervix will develop chlamydial pneumonitis within 1 to 3 months?

a. 1
b. 10
c. 50
d. 90

59–36. What is the best treatment for chlamydial cervicitis in pregnancy?

a. erythromycin estolate 250 mg po qid × 4 days
b. tetracycline 500 mg po qid × 7 days
c. erythromycin base 500 mg po qid × 7 days
d. quinolones 500 mg po qid × 14 days

59–37. What is the cure rate for chlamydial infections in pregnancy treated with azithromycin?

a. 25%
b. 50%
c. 75%
d. 95%

59–38. Lymphogranuloma venereum is difficult to differentiate from which of the following?

a. chancroid
b. granuloma inguinale
c. herpes
d. syphilis

59–39. Nongenital herpes virus infections are generally owing to which of the following?

a. HSV 1
b. HSV 2
c. HSV 6
d. all of the above

59–40. What is the average incubation time for primary herpes?

a. <1 day
b. 3 to 6 days
c. ~14 days
d. 28 to 30 days

59–41. How long does it take for all signs and symptoms of primary herpes to resolve?

a. <3 days
b. 4 to 7 days
c. 14 to 28 days
d. >42 days

59–42. Which of the following is the "gold standard" for the diagnosis of herpes?

a. tissue culture
b. ELISA tests/serology
c. DNA probes
d. cytological examination

59–43. What percentage of pregnant women will have more than one symptomatic herpes recurrence during pregnancy?

a. 20
b. 40
c. 60
d. 80

59–44. What is the most common means for acquisition of neonatal herpes virus infection?

a. transplacental
b. across intact fetal membranes
c. contact at delivery
d. postnatally

59–45. What is the risk of neonatal infection with primary maternal infection during labor?

a. <1%
b. 5%
c. 20%
d. 50%

59–46. What is the risk of neonatal herpes infection with recurrent maternal infection during labor?

a. 5%
b. 15%
c. 25%
d. 50%

59–47. What percentage of women will have a positive herpes culture during labor?

a. <0.02
b. 0.2
c. 2
d. 20

59–48. Which of the following is the recommended antepartum management scheme for prevention of neonatal herpes?

a. thorough examination intrapartum; no lesions, no cesarean section
b. weekly HSV cultures beginning at 32 weeks' gestation; cesarean section for positive culture
c. amniocentesis to exclude intra-amnionic herpes infection
d. cesarean section performed only for obstetrical indications

59–49. What type of virus is the human immuno-deficiency virus (HIV)?

    a. RNA virus
    b. DNA virus
    c. RNA retrovirus
    d. DNA retrovirus

59–50. How often is HIV infection responsible for death in women aged 25 to 44 years?

    a. 10th leading cause
    b. 5th leading cause
    c. 3rd leading cause
    d. most common cause

59–51. What is the major mode of transmission of HIV-1?

    a. fecal–oral
    b. parenterally
    c. sexual transmission
    d. perinatally

59–52. What percentage of AIDS cases in women can be attributed to heterosexual contact?

    a. 10
    b. 33
    c. 50
    d. 75

59–53. What is the median survival time for the acquired immunodeficiency syndrome?

    a. 2 years
    b. 5 years
    c. 10 years
    d. 20 years

59–54. What is the risk of HIV transmission of screened blood?

    a. 1 per 20,000
    b. 1 per 500,000
    c. 1 per 2 million
    d. 1 per 10 million

59–55. What is the rate of perinatal transmission of the HIV virus?

    a. 5 to 10%
    b. 15 to 18%
    c. 25 to 30%
    d. 50 to 60%

59–56. What was the rate of perinatal transmission in women given zidovudine according to the ACTG 076 protocol?

    a. 1%
    b. 8%
    c. 15%
    d. 25%

59–57. What is the risk of transmission of HIV to the newborn from breastfeeding?

    a. increased
    b. decreased
    c. remains the same
    d. unknown

59–58. At what CD_4 count cutoff is primary prophylaxis for *P. carinii* pneumonia recommended?

    a. <200
    b. <100
    c. <75
    d. <50

59–59. Management of health care workers exposed significantly to HIV-contaminated fluids includes which of the following?

    a. observation
    b. serial ELISA and zidovudine for positive tests
    c. serial CD_4 counts and zidovudine for CD_4 count < 500/µL
    d. counseling and zidovudine prophylaxis

59–60. What is the etiology of condylomata accuminata?

    a. *Treponema pallidum*
    b. human papillomavirus
    c. parvovirus
    d. *Hemophilus ducreyi*

59–61. What is the initial treatment of condylomata accuminata during pregnancy?

    a. podophyllin resin
    b. interferon
    c. trichloracetic acid
    d. 5-fluorouracil

59–62. Of the following virus types, which is associated with laryngeal papillomatosis?

   a. HPV 6
   b. HPV 16
   c. HPV 31
   d. HPV 50

59–63. What is the etiology of soft chancres?

   a. *Treponema pallidum*
   b. *Hemophilus ducreyi*

   c. *Trichomonas vaginalis*
   d. *Donovanosis*

59–64. Which of the following is a recommended treatment for *Hemophilus ducreyi* in pregnancy?

   a. ceftriaxone 250 mg IM
   b. erythromycin 250 mg bid for 3 days
   c. tetracycline 500 mg qid for 7 days
   d. azithromycin 1 g orally

Family Planning

60

Medical Contraception

60–1. Which of the following is NOT a true statement?

    a. There is no safe contraception.
    b. The lack of contraception is dangerous.
    c. Driving your automobile is safer than contraception.
    d. Women should be given a choice for contraception.

60–2. In the absence of contraception, what percentage of presumably fertile sexually active women will be pregnant?

    a. 90
    b. 75
    c. 50
    d. 40

60–3. What is the expected failure rate from Depo-Provera (injectable)?

    a. 0.03%
    b. 0.3%
    c. 1.0%
    d. 3.0%

60–4. What is the mechanism of action of oral contraceptives?

    a. prevent ovulation
    b. suppress gonadotropin-releasing factors
    c. suppress FSH and LH
    d. all of the above

60–5. Which of the following estrogens is used in oral contraceptives?

    a. estrone
    b. estradiol
    c. estriol
    d. equilin

60–6. What is the conversion factor for potency of ethinyl estradiol to mestranol?

    a. 1.0 to 1.0
    b. 1.2 to 1.5
    c. 2.1 to 2.3
    d. 0.4 to 0.5

60–7. What is the progestin with the least androgenic effect?

    a. norethindrone
    b. norgestrel
    c. levonorgestrel
    d. norgestimate

60–8. What is the progestin with the most estrogenic effect?

a. norgestrel
b. norethindrone
c. norethindrone acetate
d. ethynodiol diacetate

60–9. Which of the following drugs may decrease the effectiveness of oral contraceptives?

a. aspirin
b. erythromycin
c. rifampin
d. propranolol

60–10. Which of the following vitamins increases the bioavailability of ethinyl estradiol?

a. vitamin A
b. vitamin B
c. vitamin C
d. vitamin K

60–11. Which of the following is NOT reduced with oral contraceptive use?

a. menstrual blood loss
b. salpingitis
c. endometrial cancer
d. cervical cancer

60–12. In a patient taking oral contraceptives, which of the following is reduced?

a. plasma thyroxine
b. plasma cortisol
c. T_3 resin uptake
d. transcortin

60–13. Which oral contraceptive preparation likely would have the least detrimental effect on lipoproteins?

a. Ovral
b. Lo Ovral
c. Triphasil
d. Ortho Novum 7/7/7

60–14. Which of the following progestins has the greatest antagonizing effect on insulin and glucose metabolism?

a. norgesterol
b. norethindrone
c. L-norgesterol
d. ethyinodiol diacetate

60–15. The risk of cervical (preinvasive) cancer increases after how many years of oral contraceptive use?

a. 1 year
b. 3 years
c. 5 years
d. 10 years

60–16. The enzyme that enhances tryptophan metabolism (i.e., tryptophan oxygenase) is induced by which of the following?

a. estrogen
b. progesterone
c. prolactin
d. oxytocin

60–17. What is the effect of oral contraceptives on the incidence of deep venous thrombosis and embolism?

a. decreased incidence
b. does not effect the incidence
c. increases the incidence
d. increases thrombosis but not pulmonary embolism

60–18. In regard to hypertension and the use of oral contraceptives, which is NOT true?

a. Pregnancy-induced hypertension is associated with subsequent oral contraceptive hypertension.
b. Hypertension is likely related to the estrogen.
c. From 5 to 6 percent will develop hypertension on oral contraceptives.
d. Progestin-only formulations do not cause hypertension.

60–19. The current information regarding the association of myocardial infarction and oral contraceptive use suggests which of the following?

a. Low-dose pills are not associated with an increased risk to nonsmokers.
b. Low-dose pills are associated with an increased risk to nonsmokers.
c. The prostacyclin-to-thromboxane ratio shifts toward prostacyclin.
d. Platelet-activating factor is decreased in pill users who smoke.

60–20. Oral contraceptives have been reported to cause which of the following congenital defects?

    a. limb-reduction defects
    b. sexual ambiguity
    c. heart defects
    d. no association with any defects

60–21. Which is true concerning the risk of dying while using the "pill" (oral contraceptives) to a woman under 35 years of age?

    a. less than that of pregnancy
    b. greater than that of pregnancy
    c. not affected by smoking
    d. not dose related

60–22. Of the following, which is NOT an absolute contraindication to oral contraceptives?

    a. prior thromboembolism
    b. history of liver tumor on oral contraceptives previously
    c. migraine headaches
    d. breast carcinoma with positive estrogen receptors

60–23. What is the contraceptive dosage of Depo-Provera?

    a. 50 mg every 3 months
    b. 100 mg every 3 months
    c. 150 mg every 3 months
    d. 200 mg every 3 months

60–24. What is the release rate of levonorgestrel in Norplant at 60 months?

    a. 2.5 µg/d
    b. 25 µg/d
    c. 250 µg/d
    d. 2500 µg/d

60–25. What is the mechanism of action of RU 486?

    a. prevents conversion of pregnenolone to progesterone
    b. blocks or competes for progesterone receptor sites
    c. prevents LH surge
    d. facilitates prostaglandin production

60–26. Of the following, which is NOT an approved drug for postcoital contraception?

    a. ethinyl estradiol
    b. diethylstilbestrol
    c. danazol
    d. Norplant

$\boxed{61}$

Mechanical Methods of Contraception

61–1. Why were the Lippes Loop and the Cu-7 withdrawn from the market?

    a. Infections were unacceptable.
    b. Utilization was low.
    c. The cost of defense litigation was excessive.
    d. Effectiveness was unacceptable.

61–2. How often does the Progestasert need to be replaced?

    a. each year
    b. every 2 years
    c. every 3 years
    d. every 4 years

61–3. How much progesterone is supplied into the uterus daily with a Progestersert IUD?

    a. 1 μg
    b. 30 μg
    c. 65 μg
    d. 100 μg

61–4. How often does the levonorgestrel IUD need to be replaced?

    a. yearly
    b. every 2 years
    c. every 5 years
    d. every 7 years

61–5. Which of the following is NOT a mechanism of action of the intrauterine device?

    a. accelerated tubal motility
    b. prevention of ovulation
    c. local inflammatory reaction
    d. prevention of implantation

61–6. Which device is associated with the least menstrual blood loss?

    a. Cu-T 380 A
    b. Lippes Loop
    c. Cu-7
    d. Progestasert

61–7. What is the most appropriate therapy for a woman 8 weeks' pregnant with the string of a Cu-T 380 A visible at the cervix?

    a. antibiotics
    b. abortion
    c. removal of intrauterine device
    d. no therapy

61–8. What percentage of women have their IUD removed because of menorrhagia?

    a. 5
    b. 15
    c. 30
    d. 50

61–9. What is the incidence of actinomyces-like structures identified by Pap smears in women with IUDs?

    a. 0.1%
    b. 1.0 to 2.0%
    c. 6.0 to 7.0%
    d. 11.0 to 12.0%

61–10. Which of the following is NOT an absolute contraindication to using an intrauterine device?

    a. active or recent salpingitis
    b. pregnancy
    c. undiagnosed uterine bleeding
    d. uterine leiomyomata

61–11. How long should the Copper T 300 be left in the uterus?

    a. 1 year
    b. 3 years
    c. 5 years
    d. 10 years

61–12. What is the breakage rate of the female condom?

    a. 0.6%
    b. 1.0 to 2.0%
    c. 3.0 to 5.0%
    d. 8.0 to 10.0%

61–13. When is the maximal effectiveness of spermicides?

    a. the first hour after insertion
    b. equal for 6 hours
    c. equal for 8 hours
    d. equal for 24 hours

61–14. Of the following, which is increased when spermicides are used?

    a. neural tube defects
    b. limb reduction defect
    c. Down syndrome
    d. none of the above

61–15. How long after intercourse should the diaphragm remain in place?

    a. 6 hr
    b. 12 hr
    c. 18 hr
    d. 24 hr

61–16. In general, when does ovulation occur?

    a. 14 days after the last menses
    b. 14 days prior to the onset of menses
    c. 21 days after the last menses
    d. 28 days after the last menses

61–17. Which of the following has the highest accidental pregnancy rate during its first year of use?

    a. withdrawal
    b. male condom
    c. female condom
    d. progestin-only pill

62

Surgical Contraception

62–1. What is the most popular form of contraception in the United States?

    a. condoms
    b. oral contraceptives
    c. intrauterine devices
    d. sterilization

62–2. Which tubal sterilization procedure is the least likely to fail?

    a. Pomeroy
    b. Irving
    c. Parkland
    d. fimbriectomy

62–3. What is the greatest failure rate for a Parkland-type tubal sterilization?

    a. 1 in 100
    b. 1 in 200
    c. 1 in 400
    d. 1 in 1000

62–4. What is the least effective sterilization procedure?

    a. fimbriectomy
    b. Madlener
    c. Parkland
    d. Irving

62–5. With laparoscopic tubal sterilization, which factor increases morbidity?

    a. obesity
    b. previous abdominal or pelvic surgery
    c. diabetes
    d. all of the above

62–6. What is the mortality rate directly related to female sterilization?

    a. 1 in 100,000
    b. 4 in 100,000
    c. 1 in 10,000
    d. 4 in 10,000

62–7. In regard to tubal sterilization failures, which of the following is NOT true?

    a. There is fistula formation.
    b. Mechanical devices are improperly placed.
    c. With the bipolar method there is inadequate coagulation.
    d. All are preventable.

62–8. Which of the following is most likely to occur following tubal sterilization?

    a. increased blood loss with menses
    b. unchanged blood loss with menses
    c. luteal phase dysfunction
    d. ovarian varicosities

62–9. What is the success rate in microsurgical reanastomosis of a tubal sterilization secondary to Pomeroy technique?

    a. 25%
    b. 43%
    c. 59%
    d. 88%

62–10. What is the overall mortality rate from hysterectomy?

    a. 1 in 100,000
    b. 20 in 100,000
    c. 60 in 100,000
    d. 100 in 100,000

62–11. What is the failure rate of vasectomy?

    a. 1 in 100
    b. 1 in 200
    c. 1 in 300
    d. 1 in 400

62–12. Which of the following is true concerning an open-ended vasectomy?

    a. leaves the testicular end of the vas patent
    b. decreases congestive epididymitis
    c. allows a higher success rate with reanastomosis
    d. all of the above

62–13. Following a vasectomy, which statement is true?

    a. Autoimmune diseases are more common.
    b. Arteriosclerosis is accelerated.
    c. Sterility is not immediate.
    d. Testicular cancer is increased.

ANSWERS

2-24. a (*p. 26*)

2-25. c (*p. 27*)

2-26. d (*p. 29*)

2-27. c (*p. 29*)

2-28. a (*p. 30*)

2-29. c (*p. 30*)

2-30. c (*p. 30*)

2-31. a (*p. 31*)

2-32. c (*p. 31*)

2-33. a (*p. 31*)

2-34. c (*p. 31*)

2-35. c (*p. 33*)

2-36. a (*p. 20*)

CHAPTER 3

3-1. b (*p. 37*)

3-2. d (*p. 38*)

3-3. a (*p. 38*)

3-4. b (*p. 39*)

3-5. b (*p. 40*)

3-6. c (*p. 43*)

3-7. a (*p. 41*)

3-8. c (*p. 41*)

3-9. d (*p. 43*)

3-10. a (*p. 43*)

3-11. b (*p. 43*)

3-12. d (*p. 43*)

3-13. d (*p. 43*)

3-14. c (*p. 43*)

3-15. b (*p. 45*)

3-16. d (*p. 45*)

3-17. c (*p. 46*)

3-18. b (*p. 47*)

3-19. a (*p. 48*)

3-20. d (*p. 51*)

3-21. b (*p. 52*)

3-22. a (*p. 52*)

3-23. b (*p. 54*)

3-24. b (*p. 56*)

3-25. b (*p. 58*)

3-26. a (*p. 59*)

3-27. d (*p. 59*)

3-28. b (*p. 59*)

3-29. c (*p. 59*)

3-30. b (*p. 59*)

3-31. c (*p. 61*)

3-32. d (*p. 61*)

3-33. d (*p. 62*)

3-34. b (*p. 62*)

3-35. c (*p. 62*)

3-36. d (*p. 62*)

3-37. b (*p. 64*)

3–38. **d** (*p. 64*)

3–39. **a** (*p. 63*)

3–40. **c** (*p. 64*)

3–41. **d** (*p. 63*)

3–42. **d** (*p. 64*)

3–43. **b** (*p. 62*)

3–44. **d** (*p. 66*)

3–45. **c** (*p. 66*)

3–46. **b** (*p. 66*)

3–47. **d** (*p. 59*)

3–48. **c** (*p. 60*)

CHAPTER 4

4–1. **a** (*p. 71*)

4–2. **d** (*p. 71*)

4–3. **d** (*p. 72*)

4–4. **a** (*p. 72*)

4–5. **b** (*p. 72*)

4–6. **b** (*p. 75*)

4–7. **d** (*p. 78*)

4–8. **d** (*p. 79*)

4–9. **a** (*p. 79*)

4–10. **d** (*p. 80*)

4–11. **c** (*p. 75*)

4–12. **c** (*p. 81*)

4–13. **c** (*p. 83*)

4–14. **b** (*p. 84*)

4–15. **c** (*p. 85*)

4–16. **b** (*p. 85*)

4–17. **c** (*p. 86*)

4–18. **c** (*p. 88*)

4–19. **b** (*p. 90*)

4–20. **b** (*p. 73*)

4–21. **c** (*p. 75*)

4–22. **d** (*p. 75*)

4–23. **c** (*p. 77*)

CHAPTER 5

5–1. **a** (*p. 96*)

5–2. **b** (*p. 96*)

5–3. **c** (*p. 98*)

5–4. **a** (*p. 98*)

5–5. **b** (*p. 99*)

5–6. **a** (*p. 107*)

5–7. **c** (*p. 96*)

5–8. **b** (*p. 97*)

5–9. **d** (*p. 99*)

5–10. **b** (*p. 121*)

5–11. **c** (*p. 108*)

5–12. **a** (*p. 108*)

5–13. **a** (*p. 108*)

5–14. **c** (*p. 109*)

5–15. a (*p. 109*)

5–16. b (*p. 109*)

5–17. d (*p. 109*)

5–18. d (*p. 101*)

5–19. d (*p. 114*)

5–20. a (*p. 114*)

5–21. c (*p. 121*)

CHAPTER 6

6–1. d (*p. 126*)

6–2. c (*p. 126*)

6–3. a (*p. 127*)

6–4. b (*p. 128*)

6–5. d (*p. 128*)

6–6. c (*p. 128*)

6–7. d (*p. 128*)

6–8. a (*p. 129*)

6–9. c (*p. 126*)

6–10. b (*p. 130*)

6–11. d (*p. 130*)

6–12. a (*p. 130*)

6–13. d (*p. 130*)

6–14. a (*p. 131*)

6–15. c (*p. 131*)

6–16. a (*p. 139*)

6–17. d (*p. 135*)

6–18. d (*p. 135*)

6–19. d (*p. 137*)

6–20. d (*p. 138*)

6–21. c (*p. 138*)

6–22. a (*p. 139*)

6–23. c (*p. 140*)

6–24. b (*p. 142*)

6–25. a (*p. 142*)

6–26. b (*p. 141*)

6–27. b (*p. 145*)

6–28. b (*p. 144*)

6–29. d (*p. 146*)

CHAPTER 7

7–1. c (*p. 151*)

7–2. a (*p. 151*)

7–3. c (*p. 152*)

7–4. c (*p. 154*)

7–5. c (*p. 154*)

7–6. b (*p. 154*)

7–7. b (*p. 154*)

7–8. c (*p. 154*)

7–9. c (*p. 155*)

7–10. b (*p. 155*)

7–11. d (*p. 155*)

7–12. c (*p. 156*)

7–13. **d** (*p. 156*)

7–14. **c** (*p. 156*)

7–15. **a** (*p. 156*)

7–16. **b** (*p. 156*)

7–17. **c** (*p. 157*)

7–18. **b** (*p. 159*)

7–19. **a** (*p. 159*)

7–20. **b** (*p. 160*)

7–21. **c** (*p. 160*)

7–22. **b** (*p. 160*)

7–23. **a** (*p. 160*)

7–24. **a** (*p. 160*)

7–25. **c** (*p. 161*)

7–26. **b** (*p. 163*)

7–27. **a** (*p. 163*)

7–28. **d** (*p. 163*)

7–29. **a** (*p. 163*)

7–30. **d** (*p. 164*)

7–31. **c** (*p. 165*)

7–32. **b** (*p. 164*)

7–33. **b** (*p. 166*)

7–34. **d** (*p. 166*)

7–35. **b** (*p. 167*)

7–36. **b** (*p. 167*)

7–37. **c** (*p. 168*)

7–38. **a** (*p. 168*)

7–39. **d** (*p. 168*)

7–40. **c** (*p. 169*)

7–41. **b** (*p. 169*)

7–42. **c** (*p. 169*)

7–43. **c** (*p. 170*)

7–44. **b** (*p. 170*)

7–45. **c** (*p. 171*)

7–46. **b** (*p. 171*)

7–47. **a** (*p. 173*)

7–48. **d** (*p. 174*)

7–49. **c** (*p. 174*)

7–50. **d** (*p. 175*)

7–51. **c** (*p. 175*)

7–52. **a** (*p. 176*)

7–53. **d** (*p. 177*)

7–54. **a** (*p. 177*)

7–55. **a** (*p. 178*)

7–56. **b** (*p. 179*)

7–57. **c** (*p. 181*)

7–58. **c** (*p. 181*)

7–59. **d** (*p. 182*)

7–60. **c** (*p. 183*)

7–61. **d** (*p. 184*)

CHAPTER 8

8–1. **d** (*p. 191*)

8–2. **c** (*p. 192*)

8–3. **a** (*p. 194*)

8–4. **d** (*p. 194*)

8–5. **c** (*p. 195*)

8–6. **a** (*p. 195*)

8–7. **b** (*p. 196*)

8–8. **a** (*p. 197*)

8–9. **c** (*p. 197*)

8–10. **c** (*p. 197*)

8–11. **c** (*p. 198*)

8–12. **d** (*p. 198*)

8–13. **b** (*p. 198*)

8–14. **b** (*p. 200*)

8–15. **b** (*p. 200*)

8–16. **c** (*p. 201*)

8–17. **a** (*p. 201*)

8–18. **c** (*p. 201*)

8–19. **c** (*p. 201*)

8–20. **a** (*p. 201*)

8–21. **c** (*p. 202*)

8–22. **a** (*p. 203*)

8–23. **c** (*p. 203*)

8–24. **b** (*p. 203*)

8–25. **c** (*p. 203*)

8–26. **d** (*p. 204*)

8–27. **c** (*p. 205*)

8–28. **d** (*p. 205*)

8–29. **c** (*p. 206*)

8–30. **a** (*p. 206*)

8–31. **a** (*p. 206*)

8–32. **b** (*p. 207*)

8–33. **d** (*p. 207*)

8–34. **d** (*p. 207*)

8–35. **d** (*p. 207*)

8–36. **c** (*p. 208*)

8–37. **b** (*p. 208*)

8–38. **c** (*p. 210*)

8–39. **d** (*p. 210*)

8–40. **d** (*p. 211*)

8–41. **b** (*p. 212*)

8–42. **c** (*p. 214*)

8–43. **b** (*p. 215*)

8–44. **a** (*p. 217*)

8–45. **d** (*p. 217*)

8–46. **b** (*p. 218*)

8–47. **b** (*p. 219*)

8–48. **a** (*p. 219*)

8–49. **b** (*p. 220*)

8–50. **d** (*p. 205*)

8–51. b (*p. 205*)

8–52. a (*p. 208*)

CHAPTER 9

9–1. b (*p. 227*)

9–2. b (*p. 227*)

9–3. b (*p. 229*)

9–4. c (*p. 229*)

9–5. a (*p. 229*)

9–6. d (*p. 229*)

9–7. a (*p. 230*)

9–8. c (*p. 230*)

9–9. d (*p. 231*)

9–10. c (*p. 231*)

9–11. c (*p. 232*)

9–12. c (*p. 233*)

9–13. c (*p. 232*)

9–14. d (*p. 233*)

9–15. b (*p. 234*)

9–16. b (*p. 234*)

9–17. c (*p. 234*)

9–18. c (*p. 235*)

9–19. b (*p. 235*)

9–20. d (*p. 236*)

9–21. a (*p. 236*)

9–22. c (*p. 237*)

9–23. a (*p. 237*)

9–24. d (*p. 237*)

9–25. c (*p. 237*)

9–26. c (*p. 237*)

9–27. d (*p. 237*)

9–28. a (*p. 237*)

9–29. d (*p. 237*)

9–30. b (*p. 237*)

9–31. c (*p. 238*)

9–32. c (*p. 238*)

9–33. c (*p. 239*)

9–34. d (*p. 239*)

9–35. a (*p. 240*)

9–36. a (*p. 241*)

9–37. d (*p. 241*)

9–38. d (*p. 242*)

9–39. d (*p. 243*)

9–40. b (*p. 243*)

9–41. c (*p. 243*)

9–42. c (*p. 243*)

9–43. a (*p. 243*)

9–44. b (*p. 243*)

9–45. a (*p. 243*)

9–46. b (*p. 244*)

9–47. d (*p. 246*)

CHAPTER 10

10–1. b (*p. 251*)

10–2. d (*p. 251*)

10–3. b (*p. 251*)

10–4. a (*p. 251*)

10–5. d (*p. 251*)

10–6. c (*p. 251*)

10–7. c (*p. 253*)

10–8. a (*p. 253*)

10–9. b (*p. 253*)

10–10. c (*p. 253*)

10–11. c (*p. 255*)

10–12. a (*p. 255*)

10–13. b (*p. 255*)

10–14. d (*p. 257*)

10–15. a (*p. 259*)

CHAPTER 11

11–1. b (*p. 262*)

11–2. d (*p. 261*)

11–3. b (*p. 262*)

11–4. a (*p. 262*)

11–5. c (*p. 263*)

11–6. d (*p. 274*)

11–7. d (*p. 266*)

11–8. d (*p. 263*)

11–9. c (*p. 263*)

11–10. a (*p. 265*)

11–11. b (*p. 265*)

11–12. d (*p. 267*)

11–13. a (*p. 268*)

11–14. a (*p. 269*)

11–15. c (*p. 271*)

11–16. c (*p. 273*)

11–17. c (*p. 274*)

11–18. b (*p. 273*)

11–19. d (*p. 277*)

11–20. b (*p. 275*)

11–21. c (*p. 278*)

11–22. b (*p. 278*)

11–23. d (*p. 294*)

11–24. a (*p. 283*)

11–25. d (*p. 281*)

11–26. b (*p. 281*)

11–27. a (*p. 287*)

11–28. d (*p. 281*)

11–29. c (*p. 286*)

11–30. b (*p. 288*)

11–31. **a** (*p. 286*)

11–32. **a** (*p. 287*)

11–33. **d** (*p. 288*)

11–34. **a** (*p. 291*)

11–35. **d** (*p. 304*)

11–36. **c** (*p. 294*)

11–37. **a** (*p. 294*)

11–38. **d** (*p. 295*)

11–39. **c** (*p. 296*)

11–40. **a** (*p. 297*)

11–41. **a** (*p. 300*)

11–42. **b** (*p. 300*)

11–43. **a** (*p. 300*)

11–44. **b** (*p. 296*)

11–45. **d** (*p. 303*)

11–46. **d** (*p. 303*)

11–47. **d** (*p. 303*)

11–48. **d** (*p. 305*)

11–49. **a** (*p. 306*)

11–50. **c** (*p. 309*)

11–51. **a** (*p. 309*)

11–52. **c** (*p. 309*)

11–53. **d** (*p. 310*)

11–54. **b** (*p. 310*)

11–55. **d** (*p. 310*)

11–56. **c** (*p. 309*)

11–57. **c** (*p. 262*)

11–58. **d** (*p. 262*)

CHAPTER 12

12–1. **d** (*p. 319*)

12–2. **d** (*p. 319*)

12–3. **a** (*p. 319*)

12–4. **a** (*p. 319*)

12–5. **c** (*p. 320*)

12–6. **c** (*p. 321*)

12–7. **a** (*p. 321*)

12–8. **b** (*p. 325*)

12–9. **b** (*p. 321*)

12–10. **c** (*p. 324*)

12–11. **a** (*p. 322*)

12–12. **c** (*p. 321*)

12–13. **c** (*p. 325*)

12–14. **b** (*p. 325*)

12–15. **d** (*p. 325*)

CHAPTER 13

13–1. **c** (*p. 327*)

13–2. **c** (*p. 327*)

13–3. **c** (*p. 328*)

13–4. **d** (*p. 328*)

13–5. a (*p. 328*)

13–6. b (*p. 329*)

13–7. b (*p. 330*)

13–8. d (*p. 330*)

13–9. b (*p. 330*)

13–10. c (*p. 330*)

13–11. a (*p. 330*)

13–12. c (*p. 332*)

13–13. c (*p. 332*)

13–14. b (*p. 333*)

13–15. b (*p. 334*)

13–16. d (*p. 336*)

13–17. d (*p. 338*)

13–18. d (*p. 338*)

13–19. a (*p. 340*)

13–20. b (*p. 340*)

13–21. b (*p. 340*)

13–22. b (*p. 341*)

13–23. a (*p. 341*)

13–24. b (*p. 341*)

13–25. d (*p. 342*)

13–26. a (*p. 342*)

13–27. c (*p. 342*)

13–28. d (*p. 343*)

13–29. a (*p. 343*)

13–30. c (*p. 343*)

CHAPTER 14

14–1. d (*p. 347*)

14–2. c (*p. 348*)

14–3. b (*p. 348*)

14–4. b (*p. 349*)

14–5. c (*p. 350*)

14–6. b (*p. 350*)

14–7. b (*p. 351*)

14–8. c (*p. 351*)

14–9. d (*p. 351*)

14–10. d (*p. 351*)

14–11. d (*p. 351*)

14–12. b (*p. 352*)

14–13. b (*p. 352*)

14–14. c (*p. 352*)

14–15. b (*p. 356*)

14–16. b (*p. 356*)

14–17. d (*p. 357*)

14–18. a (*p. 357*)

14–19. b (*p. 357*)

14–20. c (*p. 359*)

14–21. c (*p. 359*)

14–22. d (*p. 361*)

14–23. d (*p. 360*)

14–24. c (*p. 362*)

14–25. b (*p. 366*)

14–26. **b** (*p. 367*)

14–27. **c** (*p. 369*)

14–28. **d** (*p. 371*)

14–29. **a** (*p. 372*)

14–30. **b** (*p. 373*)

14–31. **c** (*p. 373*)

14–32. **c** (*p. 374*)

CHAPTER 15

15–1. **b** (*p. 379*)

15–2. **d** (*p. 379*)

15–3. **b** (*p. 380*)

15–4. **d** (*p. 380*)

15–5. **c** (*p. 380*)

15–6. **a** (*p. 380*)

15–7. **c** (*p. 381*)

15–8. **b** (*p. 381*)

15–9. **b** (*p. 381*)

15–10. **b** (*p. 381*)

15–11. **d** (*p. 382*)

15–12. **b** (*p. 382*)

15–13. **a** (*p. 382*)

15–14. **c** (*p. 383*)

15–15. **b** (*p. 383*)

15–16. **c** (*p. 383*)

15–17. **b** (*p. 384*)

15–18. **a** (*p. 384*)

15–19. **c** (*p. 384*)

15–20. **c** (*p. 386*)

15–21. **d** (*p. 386*)

15–22. **d** (*p. 387*)

15–23. **a** (*p. 387*)

15–24. **c** (*p. 387*)

15–25. **c** (*p. 388*)

15–26. **a** (*p. 390*)

15–27. **b** (*p. 391*)

15–28. **b** (*p. 392*)

15–29. **b** (*p. 393*)

15–30. **c** (*p. 396*)

15–31. **a** (*p. 396*)

CHAPTER 16

16–1. **b** (*p. 399*)

16–2. **a** (*p. 399*)

16–3. **d** (*p. 399*)

16–4. **b** (*p. 400*)

16–5. **a** (*p. 400*)

16–6. **d** (*p. 400*)

16–7. **b** (*p. 401*)

16–8. **d** (*p. 402*)

16–9. **d** (*p. 401*)

16–10. **d** (*p. 401*)

16–11. b (*p. 402*)

16–12. d (*p. 402*)

16–13. d (*p. 402*)

16–14. b (*p. 402*)

16–15. c (*p. 403*)

16–16. b (*p. 403*)

16–17. a (*p. 403*)

16–18. c (*p. 404*)

16–19. d (*p. 405*)

16–20. c (*p. 406*)

16–21. d (*p. 407*)

16–22. d (*p. 409*)

16–23. b (*p. 410*)

CHAPTER 17

17–1. d (*p. 415*)

17–2. d (*p. 415*)

17–3. c (*p. 416*)

17–4. b (*p. 417*)

17–5. b (*p. 417*)

17–6. d (*p. 417*)

17–7. b (*p. 417*)

17–8. b (*p. 415*)

17–9. a (*p. 416*)

17–10. c (*p. 417*)

17–11. b (*p. 418*)

17–12. d (*p. 419*)

17–13. a (*p. 421*)

17–14. c (*p. 421*)

17–15. c (*p. 421*)

17–16. b (*p. 423*)

17–17. b (*p. 419*)

17–18. a (*p. 419*)

17–19. b (*p. 429*)

17–20. a (*p. 426*)

17–21. d (*p. 426*)

17–22. d (*p. 422*)

17–23. b (*p. 423*)

17–24. d (*p. 421*)

17–25. c (*p. 427*)

17–26. b (*p. 422*)

17–27. d (*p. 429*)

17–28. c (*p. 419*)

17–29. d (*p. 431*)

17–30. a (*p. 431*)

CHAPTER 18

18–1. b (*p. 435*)

18–2. d (*p. 435*)

18–3. b (*p. 435*)

18–4. a (*p. 435*)

18–5. c (*p. 435*)

18–6. b (*p. 435*)

18–7. c (*p. 435*)

18–8. a (*p. 435*)

18–9. c (*p. 438*)

18–10. b (*p. 438*)

18–11. c (*p. 439*)

18–12. d (*p. 442*)

18–13. c (*p. 442*)

18–14. d (*p. 443*)

18–15. a (*p. 443*)

18–16. c (*p. 443*)

18–17. b (*p. 443*)

18–18. c (*p. 443*)

18–19. b (*p. 445*)

18–20. b (*p. 446*)

18–21. c (*p. 447*)

18–22. b (*p. 448*)

18–23. b (*p. 447*)

18–24. b (*p. 449*)

18–25. c (*p. 450*)

18–26. b (*p. 451*)

18–27. b (*p. 455*)

18–28. d (*p. 436*)

CHAPTER 19

19–1. c (*p. 461*)

19–2. c (*p. 461*)

19–3. c (*p. 461*)

19–4. b (*p. 461*)

19–5. a (*p. 462*)

19–6. d (*p. 464*)

19–7. d (*p. 464*)

19–8. d (*p. 464*)

19–9. b (*p. 464*)

19–10. c (*p. 467*)

19–11. c (*p. 467*)

19–12. a (*p. 467*)

19–13. a (*p. 468*)

19–14. b (*p. 468*)

19–15. a (*p. 469*)

CHAPTER 20

20–1. d (*p. 473*)

20–2. b (*p. 473*)

20–3. a (*p. 474*)

20–4. b (*p. 474*)

20–5. c (*p. 474*)

20–6. a (*p. 474*)

20–7. d (*p. 475*)

20–8. a (*p. 476*)

20–9. b (*p. 476*)

20–10. d (*p. 476*)

20–11. b (*p. 476*)

20–12. c (*p. 476*)

20–13. a (*p. 476*)

20–14. c (*p. 476*)

20–15. d (*p. 476*)

20–16. b (*p. 477*)

20–17. b (*p. 477*)

20–18. a (*p. 477*)

20–19. d (*p. 478*)

20–20. d (*p. 481*)

20–21. b (*p. 482*)

20–22. d (*p. 484*)

20–23. a (*p. 483*)

20–24. c (*p. 485*)

20–25. b (*p. 485*)

20–26. d (*p. 490*)

20–27. a (*p. 490*)

20–28. d (*p. 490*)

20–29. d (*p. 492*)

CHAPTER 21

21–1. b (*p. 495*)

21–2. a (*p. 496*)

21–3. d (*p. 497*)

21–4. c (*p. 498*)

21–5. c (*p. 501*)

21–6. a (*p. 501*)

21–7. c (*p. 502*)

21–8. b (*p. 502*)

21–9. b (*p. 496*)

21–10. b (*p. 501*)

21–11. c (*p. 502*)

21–12. d (*p. 495*)

21–13. a (*p. 506*)

21–14. c (*p. 505*)

21–15. d (*p. 505*)

21–16. a (*p. 506*)

CHAPTER 22

22–1. b (*p. 509*)

22–2. d (*p. 511*)

22–3. d (*p. 511*)

22–4. d (*p. 511*)

22–5. c (*p. 511*)

22–6. b (*p. 513*)

22–7. c (*p. 512*)

22–8. c (*p. 512*)

22–9. a (*p. 514*)

22–10. a (*p. 515*)

22–11. d (*p. 515*)

22–12. c (*p. 515*)

22–13. b (*p. 518*)

22–14. d (*p. 521*)

22–15. c (*p. 522*)

22–16. b (*p. 512*)

22–17. a (*p. 513*)

22–18. c (*p. 513*)

22–19. b (*p. 510*)

22–20. c (*p. 514*)

22–21. c (*p. 527*)

CHAPTER 23

23–1. c (*p. 533*)

23–2. b (*p. 533*)

23–3. c (*p. 533*)

23–4. c (*p. 534*)

23–5. d (*p. 534*)

23–6. d (*p. 535*)

23–7. d (*p. 535*)

23–8. d (*p. 535*)

23–9. a (*p. 535*)

23–10. c (*p. 536*)

23–11. b (*p. 536*)

23–12. d (*p. 536*)

23–13. d (*p. 537*)

23–14. b (*p. 537*)

23–15. a (*p. 538*)

23–16. c (*p. 538*)

23–17. b (*p. 539*)

23–18. d (*p. 539*)

23–19. c (*p. 540*)

23–20. b (*p. 540*)

23–21. d (*p. 541*)

23–22. a (*p. 541*)

23–23. d (*p. 542*)

23–24. b (*p. 542*)

23–25. d (*p. 542*)

23–26. c (*p. 543*)

23–27. c (*p. 543*)

23–28. a (*p. 543*)

CHAPTER 24

24–1. b (*p. 547*)

24–2. a (*p. 547*)

24–3. a (*p. 547*)

24–4. a (*p. 547*)

24–5. b (*p. 548*)

24–6. d (*p. 548*)

24–7. d (*p. 548*)

24–8. b (*p. 548*)

24–9. a (*p. 550*)

24–10. c (*p. 549*)

24–11. d (*p. 549*)

24–12. d (*p. 549*)

24–13. b (*p. 549*)

24–14. d (*p. 550*)

24–15. b (*p. 550*)

24–16. d (*p. 551*)

24–17. d (*p. 551*)

24–18. a (*p. 551*)

24–19. c (*p. 552*)

24–20. b (*p. 552*)

24–21. d (*p. 552*)

24–22. b (*p. 552*)

24–23. d (*p. 552*)

24–24. b (*p. 552*)

24–25. b (*p. 552*)

24–26. d (*p. 553*)

24–27. b (*p. 553*)

24–28. d (*p. 553*)

24–29. a (*p. 553*)

24–30. a (*p. 554*)

24–31. d (*p. 554*)

24–32. c (*p. 555*)

24–33. b (*p. 556*)

24–34. b (*p. 556*)

24–35. a (*p. 557*)

24–36. b (*p. 557*)

24–37. c (*p. 558*)

24–38. b (*p. 558*)

24–39. d (*p. 558*)

24–40. b (*p. 558*)

24–41. d (*p. 559*)

24–42. b (*p. 560*)

24–43. c (*p. 560*)

24–44. b (*p. 560*)

24–45. a (*p. 560*)

24–46. d (*p. 560*)

24–47. c (*p. 562*)

24–48. a (*p. 562*)

24–49. b (*p. 563*)

24–50. d (*p. 563*)

24–51. d (*p. 563*)

24–52. c (*p. 564*)

24–53. a (*p. 564*)

24–54. c (*p. 564*)

24–55. c (*p. 565*)

CHAPTER 25

25–1. b (*p. 569*)

25–2. a (*p. 570*)

25–3. b (*p. 570*)

25–4. c (*p. 570*)

25–5. d (*p. 571*)

25–6. c (*p. 571*)

25–7. c (*p. 571*)

25–8. d (*p. 571*)

25–9. a (*p. 572*)

25–10. b (*p. 573*)

25–11. c (*p. 574*)

25–12. d (*p. 574*)

25–13. c (*p. 575*)

CHAPTER 26

26–1. c (*p. 579*)

26–2. a (*p. 579*)

26–3. b (*p. 581*)

26–4. c (*p. 580*)

26–5. a (*p. 583*)

26–6. d (*p. 583*)

26–7. b (*p. 584*)

26–8. d (*p. 584*)

26–9. d (*p. 585*)

26–10. c (*p. 585*)

26–11. a (*p. 585*)

26–12. b (*p. 586*)

26–13. a (*p. 586*)

26–14. d (*p. 586*)

26–15. c (*p. 586*)

26–16. c (*p. 588*)

26–17. d (*p. 590*)

26–18. c (*p. 591*)

26–19. d (*p. 591*)

26–20. d (*p. 591*)

26–21. b (*p. 591*)

26–22. d (*p. 593*)

26–23. c (*p. 599*)

26–24. b (*p. 600*)

26–25. c (*p. 594*)

CHAPTER 27

27–1. d (*p. 607*)

27–2. b (*p. 607*)

27–3. d (*p. 607*)

27–4. d (*p. 608*)

27–5. c (*p. 608*)

27–6. a (*p. 609*)

27–7. b (*p. 610*)

27–8. b (*p. 610*)

27–9. d (*p. 611*)

27–10. b (*p. 613*)

27–11. d (*p. 614*)

27–12. c (*p. 615*)

27–13. d (*p. 615*)

27–14. b (*p. 617*)

27–15. d (*p. 622*)

27–16. c (*p. 622*)

27–17. c (*p. 622*)

27–18. b (*p. 623*)

27–19. c (*p. 624*)

27–20. d (*p. 626*)

27–21. d (*p. 627*)

27–22. d (*p. 628*)

28–20. c (*p. 651*)

28–21. c (*p. 651*)

28–22. c (*p. 651*)

28–23. c (*p. 652*)

28–24. d (*p. 652*)

28–25. c (*p. 652*)

CHAPTER 28

28–1. b (*p. 635*)

28–2. b (*p. 641*)

28–3. a (*p. 638*)

28–4. a (*p. 635*)

28–5. c (*p. 635*)

28–6. b (*p. 635*)

28–7. c (*p. 636*)

28–8. c (*p. 637*)

28–9. d (*p. 637*)

28–10. b (*p. 638*)

28–11. a (*p. 639*)

28–12. c (*p. 641*)

28–13. c (*p. 642*)

28–14. a (*p. 644*)

28–15. c (*p. 644*)

28–16. c (*p. 645*)

28–17. d (*p. 646*)

28–18. c (*p. 646*)

28–19. b (*p. 648*)

CHAPTER 29

29–1. b (*p. 657*)

29–2. c (*p. 657*)

29–3. a (*p. 657*)

29–4. c (*p. 657*)

29–5. a (*p. 658*)

29–6. d (*p. 659*)

29–7. c (*p. 659*)

29–8. c (*p. 659*)

29–9. b (*p. 659*)

29–10. d (*p. 660*)

29–11. a (*p. 661*)

29–12. b (*p. 661*)

29–13. d (*p. 662*)

29–14. c (*p. 662*)

29–15. c (*p. 662*)

29–16. c (*p. 663*)

29–17. d (*p. 663*)

29–18. c (*p. 663*)

29–19. c (*p. 664*)

29–20. d (*p. 664*)

29–21. a (*p. 664*)

29–22. a (*p. 665*)

29–23. c (*p. 664*)

CHAPTER 30

30–1. a (*p. 669*)

30–2. c (*p. 669*)

30–3. b (*p. 669*)

30–4. c (*p. 669*)

30–5. d (*p. 669*)

30–6. c (*p. 669*)

30–7. b (*p. 670*)

30–8. c (*p. 670*)

30–9. c (*p. 670*)

30–10. a (*p. 671*)

30–11. d (*p. 671*)

30–12. b (*p. 671*)

30–13. d (*p. 671*)

30–14. d (*p. 671*)

30–15. b (*p. 671*)

30–16. a (*p. 672*)

30–17. b (*p. 672*)

30–18. c (*p. 672*)

30–19. c (*p. 672*)

30–20. c (*p. 673*)

30–21. a (*p. 674*)

30–22. c (*p. 674*)

30–23. a (*p. 674*)

30–24. c (*p. 674*)

30–25. b (*p. 675*)

30–26. c (*p. 675*)

30–27. a (*p. 675*)

30–28. b (*p. 675*)

30–29. c (*p. 675*)

30–30. b (*p. 677*)

30–31. b (*p. 678*)

30–32. d (*p. 679*)

30–33. a (*p. 679*)

30–34. b (*p. 680*)

30–35. b (*p. 681*)

30–36. b (*p. 681*)

30–37. b (*p. 682*)

30–38. d (*p. 682*)

30–39. d (*p. 683*)

30–40. c (*p. 683*)

30–41. c (*p. 684*)

30–42. b (*p. 684*)

30–43. c (*p. 684*)

30–44. b (*p. 686*)

30–45. c (*p. 687*)

30–46. b (*p. 688*)

30–47. c (*p. 678*)

30–48. b (*p. 679*)

30–49. a (*p. 677*)

30–50. c (*p. 677*)

30–51. a (*p. 677*)

30–52. b (*p. 677*)

30–53. b (*p. 677*)

CHAPTER 31

31–1. d (*p. 693*)

31–2. a (*p. 694*)

31–3. c (*p. 694*)

31–4. c (*p. 695*)

31–5. b (*p. 695*)

31–6. d (*p. 695*)

31–7. c (*p. 696*)

31–8. d (*p. 696*)

31–9. b (*p. 700*)

31–10. a (*p. 700*)

31–11. c (*p. 697*)

31–12. c (*p. 698*)

31–13. d (*p. 701*)

31–14. d (*p. 701*)

31–15. b (*p. 702*)

31–16. c (*p. 701*)

31–17. d (*p. 701*)

31–18. a (*p. 703*)

31–19. b (*p. 705*)

31–20. a (*p. 705*)

31–21. d (*p. 706*)

31–22. a (*p. 707*)

31–23. c (*p. 709*)

31–24. a (*p. 710*)

31–25. a (*p. 711*)

31–26. c (*p. 712*)

31–27. c (*p. 712*)

31–28. b (*p. 712*)

31–29. d (*p. 713*)

31–30. c (*p. 714*)

31–31. c (*p. 715*)

31–32. d (*p. 706*)

31–33. a (*p. 707*)

31–34. d (*p. 708*)

31–35. c (*p. 708*)

31–36. c (*p. 716*)

31–37. d (*p. 718*)

31–38. b (*p. 722*)

31–39. c (*p. 723*)

31–40. c (*p. 722*)

31–41. c (*p. 722*)

31–42. c (*p. 723*)

31-43. a (*p. 730*)

31-44. a (*p. 731*)

31-45. b (*p. 732*)

CHAPTER 32

32-1. b (*p. 745*)

32-2. c (*p. 745*)

32-3. d (*p. 746*)

32-4. c (*p. 746*)

32-5. c (*p. 746*)

32-6. b (*p. 747*)

32-7. a (*p. 749*)

32-8. d (*p. 750*)

32-9. b (*p. 750*)

32-10. b (*p. 751*)

32-11. b (*p. 751*)

32-12. a (*p. 752*)

32-13. c (*p. 754*)

32-14. b (*p. 751*)

32-15. d (*p. 754*)

32-16. b (*p. 756*)

32-17. a (*p. 756*)

32-18. d (*p. 756*)

32-19. c (*p. 756*)

32-20. c (*p. 758*)

32-21. a (*p. 750*)

32-22. d (*p. 767*)

32-23. d (*p. 761*)

32-24. c (*p. 760*)

32-25. d (*p. 763*)

32-26. b (*p. 763*)

32-27. c (*p. 763*)

32-28. a (*p. 763*)

32-29. c (*p. 764*)

32-30. a (*p. 764*)

32-31. b (*p. 764*)

32-32. b (*p. 764*)

32-33. a (*p. 765*)

32-34. b (*p. 765*)

32-35. c (*p. 767*)

32-36. d (*p. 767*)

32-37. d (*p. 768*)

32-38. c (*p. 771*)

32-39. d (*p. 771*)

32-40. a (*p. 771*)

32-41. b (*p. 772*)

32-42. d (*p. 772*)

32-43. c (*p. 773*)

32-44. c (*p. 773*)

32-45. d (*p. 774*)

32-46. d (*p. 776*)

32-47. b (*p. 777*)

32–48. c (*p. 777*)

32–49. c (*p. 779*)

32–50. b (*p. 779*)

32–51. c (*p. 779*)

32–52. d (*p. 779*)

CHAPTER 33

33–1. b (*p. 783*)

33–2. b (*p. 783*)

33–3. d (*p. 783*)

33–4. a (*p. 783*)

33–5. b (*p. 784*)

33–6. b (*p. 784*)

33–7. b (*p. 785*)

33–8. c (*p. 785*)

33–9. a (*p. 785*)

33–10. b (*p. 786*)

33–11. b (*p. 786*)

33–12. c (*p. 786*)

33–13. a (*p. 787*)

33–14. d (*p. 787*)

33–15. c (*p. 789*)

33–16. c (*p. 789*)

33–17. a (*p. 791*)

33–18. d (*p. 792*)

33–19. a (*p. 794*)

CHAPTER 34

34–1. c (*p. 797*)

34–2. c (*p. 797*)

34–3. c (*p. 797*)

34–4. d (*p. 798*)

34–5. c (*p. 801*)

34–6. d (*p. 802*)

34–7. a (*p. 803*)

34–8. d (*p. 804*)

34–9. b (*p. 804*)

34–10. a (*p. 804*)

34–11. d (*p. 805*)

34–12. b (*p. 806*)

34–13. a (*p. 807*)

34–14. d (*p. 808*)

34–15. b (*p. 808*)

34–16. a (*p. 820*)

34–17. b (*p. 809*)

34–18. d (*p. 810*)

34–19. c (*p. 810*)

34–20. d (*p. 813*)

34–21. b (*p. 817*)

34–22. b (*p. 817*)

34–23. c (*p. 818*)

34–24. d (*p. 819*)

34–25. a (*p. 819*)

CHAPTER 35

35–1. c (*p. 827*)

35–2. c (*p. 828*)

35–3. c (*p. 828*)

35–4. b (*p. 828*)

35–5. d (*p. 828*)

35–6. b (*p. 830*)

35–7. b (*p. 828*)

35–8. c (*p. 829*)

35–9. a (*p. 830*)

35–10. c (*p. 832*)

35–11. c (*p. 833*)

35–12. d (*p. 833*)

35–13. d (*p. 830*)

CHAPTER 36

36–1. b (*p. 839*)

36–2. c (*p. 839*)

36–3. d (*p. 840*)

36–4. b (*p. 840*)

36–5. c (*p. 841*)

36–6. c (*p. 841*)

36–7. d (*p. 842*)

36–8. c (*p. 843*)

36–9. a (*p. 843*)

36–10. b (*p. 844*)

36–11. c (*p. 844*)

36–12. b (*p. 845*)

36–13. b (*p. 846*)

36–14. d (*p. 846*)

36–15. d (*p. 847*)

36–16. a (*p. 843*)

36–17. d (*p. 843*)

CHAPTER 37

37–1. c (*p. 855*)

37–2. c (*p. 855*)

37–3. b (*p. 855*)

37–4. d (*p. 856*)

37–5. a (*p. 857*)

37–6. d (*p. 858*)

CHAPTER 38

38–1. c (*p. 861*)

38–2. b (*p. 862*)

38–3. a (*p. 864*)

38–4. b (*p. 862*)

38–5. a (*p. 864*)

38–6. b (*p. 865*)

38–7. a (*p. 862*)

38–8. b (*p. 868*)

38–9. d (*p. 873*)

38–10. b (*p. 866*)

38–11. d (*p. 869*)

38–12. c (*p. 869*)

38–13. c (*p. 870*)

38–14. d (*p. 870*)

38–15. b (*p. 870*)

38–16. c (*p. 873*)

38–17. d (*p. 873*)

38–18. b (*p. 874*)

38–19. c (*p. 870*)

38–20. b (*p. 880*)

38–21. d (*p. 874*)

38–22. a (*p. 874*)

38–23. b (*p. 877*)

38–24. c (*p. 877*)

38–25. a (*p. 880*)

38–26. c (*p. 883*)

38–27. b (*p. 883*)

38–28. d (*p. 884*)

38–29. a (*p. 886*)

38–30. d (*p. 887*)

CHAPTER 39

39–1. b (*p. 895*)

39–2. d (*p. 895*)

39–3. c (*p. 895*)

39–4. c (*p. 895*)

39–5. a (*p. 896*)

39–6. a (*p. 897*)

39–7. a (*p. 898*)

39–8. d (*p. 898*)

39–9. a (*p. 898*)

39–10. c (*p. 898*)

39–11. d (*p. 899*)

39–12. b (*p. 899*)

39–13. a (*p. 900*)

39–14. a (*p. 900*)

39–15. d (*p. 900*)

39–16. a (*p. 901*)

39–17. d (*p. 902*)

39–18. c (*p. 902*)

39–19. d (*p. 902*)

39–20. b (*p. 903*)

39–21. a (*p. 902*)

39–22. d (*p. 903*)

39–23. b (*p. 903*)

39–24. d (*p. 904*)

39–25. c (*p. 904*)

39–26. c (*p. 903*)

39–27. c (*p. 903*)

39–28. d (*p. 904*)

39–29. c (*p. 904*)

39–30. **d** (*p. 905*)

39–31. **a** (*p. 905*)

39–32. **a** (*p. 905*)

39–33. **c** (*p. 905*)

39–34. **d** (*p. 905*)

39–35. **a** (*p. 905*)

39–36. **d** (*p. 906*)

39–37. **c** (*p. 907*)

39–38. **a** (*p. 907*)

39–39. **d** (*p. 908*)

39–40. **b** (*p. 908*)

39–41. **b** (*p. 908*)

39–42. **d** (*p. 909*)

39–43. **a** (*p. 909*)

39–44. **d** (*p. 909*)

39–45. **b** (*p. 909*)

39–46. **b** (*p. 909*)

39–47. **d** (*p. 909*)

39–48. **d** (*p. 910*)

39–49. **b** (*p. 912*)

39–50. **c** (*p. 913*)

CHAPTER 40

40–1. **c** (*p. 920*)

40–2. **d** (*p. 920*)

40–3. **a** (*p. 922*)

40–4. **c** (*p. 922*)

40–5. **d** (*p. 922*)

40–6. **d** (*p. 922*)

40–7. **d** (*p. 922*)

40–8. **d** (*p. 925*)

40–9. **c** (*p. 922*)

40–10. **d** (*p. 923*)

40–11. **d** (*p. 923*)

40–12. **c** (*p. 923*)

40–13. **d** (*p. 924*)

40–14. **a** (*p. 924*)

40–15. **a** (*p. 925*)

40–16. **a** (*p. 925*)

40–17. **d** (*p. 925*)

40–18. **c** (*p. 926*)

40–19. **b** (*p. 926*)

40–20. **b** (*p. 926*)

40–21. **a** (*p. 927*)

40–22. **b** (*p. 927*)

40–23. **b** (*p. 928*)

40–24. **a** (*p. 928*)

40–25. **b** (*p. 928*)

40–26. **b** (*p. 928*)

40–27. **a** (*p. 931*)

40–28. **d** (*p. 931*)

40–29. **d** (*p. 932*)

40–30. a (*p. 932*)

40–31. c (*p. 932*)

40–32. a (*p. 933*)

40–33. a (*p. 936*)

40–34. b (*p. 936*)

CHAPTER 41

41–1. b (*p. 943*)

41–2. c (*p. 943*)

41–3. c (*p. 943*)

41–4. c (*p. 943*)

41–5. d (*p. 943*)

41–6. d (*p. 943*)

41–7. b (*p. 943*)

41–8. a (*p. 944*)

41–9. a (*p. 944*)

41–10. b (*p. 944*)

41–11. b (*p. 944*)

41–12. d (*p. 944*)

41–13. b (*p. 945*)

41–14. d (*p. 946*)

41–15. a (*p. 945*)

41–16. a (*p. 946*)

41–17. b (*p. 946*)

41–18. a (*p. 946*)

41–19. d (*p. 946*)

41–20. d (*p. 946*)

41–21. c (*p. 946*)

41–22. d (*p. 947*)

41–23. d (*p. 947*)

41–24. a (*p. 947*)

41–25. c (*p. 947*)

41–26. b (*p. 948*)

41–27. b (*p. 949*)

41–28. a (*p. 949*)

41–29. c (*p. 949*)

41–30. c (*p. 949*)

41–31. d (*p. 951*)

41–32. a (*p. 952*)

41–33. c (*p. 953*)

41–34. d (*p. 953*)

41–35. b (*p. 954*)

41–36. c (*p. 955*)

41–37. c (*p. 955*)

41–38. d (*p. 956*)

41–39. b (*p. 956*)

41–40. b (*p. 956*)

41–41. a (*p. 958*)

CHAPTER 42

42–1. d (*p. 967*)

42–2. a (*p. 967*)

42–3. **d** (*p. 968*)

42–4. **a** (*p. 968*)

42–5. **b** (*p. 969*)

42–6. **c** (*p. 970*)

42–7. **b** (*p. 970*)

42–8. **c** (*p. 971*)

42–9. **d** (*p. 971*)

42–10. **c** (*p. 971*)

42–11. **c** (*p. 972*)

42–12. **d** (*p. 972*)

42–13. **b** (*p. 972*)

42–14. **d** (*p. 972*)

42–15. **c** (*p. 973*)

42–16. **a** (*p. 973*)

42–17. **d** (*p. 973*)

42–18. **b** (*p. 974*)

42–19. **c** (*p. 974*)

42–20. **d** (*p. 974*)

42–21. **d** (*p. 974*)

42–22. **a** (*p. 976*)

42–23. **c** (*p. 976*)

42–24. **b** (*p. 976*)

42–25. **b** (*p. 976*)

42–26. **d** (*p. 976*)

42–27. **a** (*p. 976*)

42–28. **a** (*p. 976*)

42–29. **d** (*p. 978*)

42–30. **c** (*p. 977*)

42–31. **c** (*p. 977*)

42–32. **d** (*p. 977*)

42–33. **d** (*p. 978*)

42–34. **a** (*p. 978*)

42–35. **d** (*p. 978*)

42–36. **d** (*p. 978*)

42–37. **c** (*p. 981*)

42–38. **c** (*p. 981*)

42–39. **a** (*p. 981*)

42–40. **c** (*p. 982*)

42–41. **a** (*p. 982*)

42–42. **a** (*p. 982*)

42–43. **d** (*p. 982*)

42–44. **c** (*p. 983*)

42–45. **d** (*p. 983*)

42–46. **c** (*p. 983*)

42–47. **a** (*p. 983*)

42–48. **a** (*p. 983*)

42–49. **b** (*p. 985*)

42–50. **b** (*p. 985*)

42–51. **c** (*p. 986*)

42–52. **b** (*p. 986*)

42–53. **b** (*p. 986*)

42–54. **d** (*p. 989*)

42–55. **d** (*p. 990*)

42–56. **d** (*p. 991*)

42–57. **a** (*p. 991*)

42–58. **d** (*p. 992*)

42–59. **b** (*p. 992*)

42–60. **c** (*p. 992*)

42–61. **c** (*p. 992*)

42–62. **b** (*p. 993*)

42–63. **a** (*p. 993*)

42–64. **a** (*p. 993*)

42–65. **d** (*p. 995*)

42–66. **c** (*p. 996*)

42–67. **c** (*p. 997*)

42–68. **a** (*p. 997*)

42–69. **a** (*p. 997*)

42–70. **b** (*p. 998*)

42–71. **c** (*p. 999*)

42–72. **b** (*p. 999*)

42–73. **d** (*p. 1000*)

42–74. **c** (*p. 1001*)

42–75. **b** (*p. 1001*)

43–4. **b** (*p. 1010*)

43–5. **a** (*p. 1010*)

43–6. **d** (*p. 1011*)

43–7. **a** (*p. 1011*)

43–8. **c** (*p. 1012*)

43–9. **c** (*p. 1012*)

43–10. **d** (*p. 1012*)

43–11. **d** (*p. 1013*)

43–12. **c** (*p. 1013*)

43–13. **a** (*p. 1013*)

43–14. **b** (*p. 1013*)

43–15. **b** (*p. 1013*)

43–16. **d** (*p. 1015*)

43–17. **d** (*p. 1015*)

43–18. **b** (*p. 1017*)

43–19. **d** (*p. 1017*)

43–20. **c** (*p. 1017*)

43–21. **b** (*p. 1018*)

43–22. **a** (*p. 1019*)

43–23. **d** (*p. 1019*)

43–24. **a** (*p. 1020*)

CHAPTER 43

43–1. **b** (*p.1009*)

43–2. **b** (*p.1009*)

43–3. **c** (*p. 1010*)

CHAPTER 44

44–1. **a** (*p. 1023*)

44–2. **c** (*p. 1023*)

44–3. **c** (*p. 1023*)

44–4. **d** (*p. 1025*)

44–5. **b** (*p. 1026*)

44–6. **b** (*p. 1027*)

44–7. **b** (*p. 1027*)

44–8. **b** (*p. 1028*)

44–9. **a** (*p. 1028*)

44–10. **a** (*p. 1029*)

44–11. **c** (*p. 1029*)

44–12. **a** (*p. 1029*)

44–13. **d** (*p. 1030*)

44–14. **a** (*p. 1030*)

44–15. **a** (*p. 1031*)

44–16. **c** (*p. 1031*)

44–17. **a** (*p. 1031*)

44–18. **c** (*p. 1032*)

44–19. **c** (*p. 1032*)

44–20. **b** (*p. 1032*)

44–21. **d** (*p. 1032*)

44–22. **b** (*p. 1033*)

44–23. **d** (*p. 1033*)

44–24. **c** (*p. 1033*)

44–25. **d** (*p. 1034*)

44–26. **c** (*p. 1034*)

44–27. **c** (*p. 1034*)

44–28. **c** (*p. 1035*)

44–29. **d** (*p. 1035*)

44–30. **c** (*p. 1036*)

44–31. **b** (*p. 1036*)

44–32. **d** (*p. 1038*)

44–33. **a** (*p. 1038*)

44–34. **a** (*p. 1038*)

44–35. **b** (*p. 1038*)

44–36. **c** (*p. 1040*)

CHAPTER 45

45–1. **a** (*p. 1046*)

45–2. **d** (*p. 1046*)

45–3. **c** (*p. 1046*)

45–4. **b** (*p. 1047*)

45–5. **b** (*p. 1050*)

45–6. **a** (*p. 1047*)

45–7. **a** (*p. 1049*)

45–8. **a** (*p. 1050*)

45–9. **b** (*p. 1050*)

45–10. **d** (*p. 1050*)

45–11. **c** (*p. 1050*)

45–12. **a** (*p. 1050*)

45–13. **c** (*p. 1050*)

45–14. **d** (*p. 1050*)

45–15. **c** (*p. 1051*)

45–16. **a** (*p. 1052*)

45–17. **b** (*p. 1053*)

45–18. **c** (*p. 1054*)

CHAPTER 46

46–1. **d** (*p. 1060*)

46–2. **b** (*p. 1061*)

46–3. **b** (*p. 1061*)

46–4. **a** (*p. 1061*)

46–5. **b** (*p. 1061*)

46–6. **b** (*p. 1061*)

46–7. **c** (*p. 1062*)

46–8. **a** (*p. 1062*)

46–9. **c** (*p. 1062*)

46–10. **d** (*p. 1063*)

46–11. **b** (*p. 1064*)

46–12. **a** (*p. 1064*)

46–13. **d** (*p. 1064*)

46–14. **d** (*p. 1065*)

46–15. **d** (*p. 1065*)

46–16. **a** (*p. 1065*)

46–17. **d** (*p. 1066*)

46–18. **c** (*p. 1066*)

46–19. **c** (*p. 1069*)

46–20. **a** (*p. 1070*)

46–21. **d** (*p. 1071*)

46–22. **a** (*p. 1071*)

46–23. **b** (*p. 1071*)

46–24. **c** (*p. 1072*)

CHAPTER 47

47–1. **b** (*p. 1079*)

47–2. **d** (*p. 1079*)

47–3. **a** (*p. 1079*)

47–4. **c** (*p. 1080*)

47–5. **d** (*p. 1080*)

47–6. **d** (*p. 1081*)

47–7. **a** (*p. 1081*)

47–8. **c** (*p. 1081*)

47–9. **b** (*p. 1082*)

47–10. **d** (*p. 1082*)

47–11. **a** (*p. 1082*)

47–12. **c** (*p. 1082*)

47–13. **c** (*p. 1083*)

47–14. **a** (*p. 1083*)

47–15. **a** (*p. 1084*)

47–16. **c** (*p. 1084*)

47–17. **d** (*p. 1084*)

47–18. **b** (*p. 1085*)

47–19. **d** (*p. 1085*)

47–20. **d** (*p. 1085*)

47–21. **b** (*p. 1085*)

47–22. **b** (*p. 1086*)

47–23. **c** (*p. 1086*)

47–24. **c** (*p. 1086*)

47–25. d (*p. 1086*)

47–26. d (*p. 1086*)

47–27. a (*p. 1087*)

47–28. c (*p. 1087*)

47–29. d (*p. 1087*)

47–30. b (*p. 1088*)

47–31. a (*p. 1088*)

47–32. c (*p. 1088*)

47–33. d (*p. 1089*)

47–34. a (*p. 1089*)

47–35. d (*p. 1089*)

47–36. a (*p. 1089*)

47–37. d (*p. 1089*)

47–38. b (*p. 1090*)

47–39. a (*p. 1090*)

47–40. d (*p. 1091*)

47–41. c (*p. 1091*)

47–42. d (*p. 1092*)

47–43. c (*p. 1092*)

47–44. b (*p. 1094*)

47–45. a (*p. 1094*)

47–46. d (*p. 1094*)

47–47. b (*p. 1095*)

47–48. b (*p. 1095*)

47–49. d (*p. 1095*)

47–50. b (*p. 1096*)

47–51. b (*p. 1096*)

47–52. c (*p. 1096*)

47–53. c (*p. 1096*)

47–54. c (*p. 1096*)

47–55. b (*p. 1096*)

47–56. d (*p. 1097*)

47–57. c (*p. 1097*)

47–58. c (*p. 1097*)

47–59. b (*p. 1098*)

CHAPTER 48

48–1. b (*p. 1103*)

48–2. b (*p. 1103*)

48–3. a (*p. 1103*)

48–4. c (*p. 1103*)

48–5. a (*p. 1104*)

48–6. d (*p. 1104*)

48–7. a (*p. 1104*)

48–8. d (*p. 1104*)

48–9. b (*p. 1105*)

48–10. d (*p. 1105*)

48–11. a (*p. 1105*)

48–12. b (*p. 1106*)

48–13. c (*p. 1106*)

48–14. b (*p. 1106*)

48–15. b (*p. 1107*)

48–16. d (*p. 1107*)

48–17. a (*p. 1107*)

48–18. d (*p. 1107*)

48–19. c (*p. 1107*)

48–20. c (*p. 1108*)

48–21. c (*p. 1108*)

48–22. a (*p. 1108*)

48–23. a (*p. 1108*)

48–24. b (*p. 1108*)

48–25. c (*p. 1109*)

48–26. d (*p. 1109*)

48–27. b (*p. 1109*)

48–28. d (*p. 1109*)

48–29. c (*p. 1109*)

48–30. a (*p. 1109*)

48–31. b (*p. 1110*)

48–32. d (*p. 1110*)

48–33. c (*p. 1110*)

48–34. b (*p. 1110*)

48–35. b (*p. 1110*)

48–36. c (*p. 1111*)

48–37. a (*p. 1112*)

48–38. a (*p. 1112*)

48–39. b (*p. 1112*)

48–40. a (*p. 1112*)

48–41. a (*p. 1112*)

48–42. c (*p. 1113*)

48–43. c (*p. 1113*)

48–44. a (*p. 1114*)

48–45. b (*p. 1114*)

48–46. c (*p. 1115*)

48–47. b (*p. 1115*)

48–48. d (*p. 1115*)

48–49. c (*p. 1116*)

48–50. a (*p. 1116*)

48–51. b (*p. 1116*)

48–52. d (*p. 1116*)

48–53. d (*p. 1117*)

48–54. b (*p. 1117*)

48–55. a (*p. 1118*)

48–56. c (*p. 1119*)

48–57. d (*p. 1119*)

48–58. a (*p. 1119*)

48–59. d (*p. 1119*)

48–60. c (*p. 1120*)

48–61. d (*p. 1120*)

48–62. a (*p. 1121*)

CHAPTER 49

49-1. d (*p. 1125*)

49-2. d (*p. 1125*)

49-3. a (*p. 1125*)

49-4. a (*p. 1126*)

49-5. b (*p. 1126*)

49-6. c (*p. 1126*)

49-7. c (*p. 1126*)

49-8. c (*p. 1128*)

49-9. d (*p. 1128*)

49-10. d (*p. 1128*)

49-11. b (*p. 1128*)

49-12. c (*p. 1128*)

49-13. a (*p. 1128*)

49-14. b (*p. 1129*)

49-15. d (*p. 1129*)

49-16. c (*p. 1130*)

49-17. d (*p. 1132*)

49-18. c (*p. 1133*)

49-19. b (*p. 1131*)

49-20. d (*p. 1132*)

49-21. b (*p. 1133*)

49-22. a (*p. 1133*)

49-23. d (*p. 1134*)

49-24. c (*p. 1134*)

49-25. c (*p. 1134*)

49-26. c (*p. 1134*)

49-27. c (*p. 1134*)

49-28. b (*p. 1134*)

49-29. a (*p. 1135*)

49-30. b (*p. 1135*)

49-31. d (*p. 1135*)

49-32. c (*p. 1135*)

49-33. d (*p. 1135*)

49-34. c (*p. 1135*)

49-35. d (*p. 1136*)

49-36. a (*p. 1136*)

49-37. b (*p. 1136*)

49-38. c (*p. 1137*)

49-39. b (*p. 1137*)

49-40. d (*p. 1138*)

49-41. c (*p. 1139*)

49-42. a (*p. 1139*)

49-43. b (*p. 1139*)

49-44. a (*p. 1139*)

49-45. b (*p. 1140*)

49-46. d (*p. 1140*)

49-47. c (*p. 1140*)

49-48. d (*p. 1141*)

CHAPTER 50

50–1. b (*p. 1145*)

50–2. b (*p. 1145*)

50–3. c (*p. 1145*)

50–4. a (*p. 1145*)

50–5. d (*p. 1147*)

50–6. a (*p. 1147*)

50–7. d (*p. 1147*)

50–8. d (*p. 1147*)

50–9. b (*p. 1147*)

50–10. c (*p. 1147*)

50–11. c (*p. 1148*)

50–12. a (*p. 1149*)

50–13. a (*p. 1148*)

50–14. b (*p. 1149*)

50–15. a (*p. 1150*)

50–16. c (*p. 1151*)

50–17. c (*p. 1151*)

50–18. d (*p. 1151*)

50–19. d (*p. 1152*)

50–20. d (*p. 1153*)

50–21. b (*p. 1154*)

50–22. a (*p. 1154*)

50–23. a (*p. 1154*)

50–24. b (*p. 1154*)

50–25. c (*p. 1154*)

50–26. b (*p. 1154*)

50–27. a (*p. 1155*)

50–28. b (*p. 1155*)

50–29. d (*p. 1156*)

50–30. b (*p. 1156*)

50–31. c (*p. 1157*)

50–32. b (*p. 1159*)

50–33. b (*p. 1160*)

50–34. b (*p. 1159*)

50–35. c (*p. 1159*)

50–36. a (*p. 1160*)

50–37. b (*p. 1160*)

50–38. d (*p. 1160*)

50–39. c (*p. 1160*)

50–40. c (*p. 1160*)

50–41. d (*p. 1161*)

50–42. c (*p. 1161*)

50–43. c (*p. 1161*)

50–44. c (*p. 1161*)

50–45. b (*p. 1162*)

50–46. b (*p. 1163*)

50–47. a (*p. 1163*)

50–48. c (*p. 1164*)

50–49. a (*p. 1164*)

50–50. b (*p. 1164*)

50–51. b (*p. 1165*)

50–52. d (*p. 1165*)

50–53. b (*p. 1165*)

50–54. c (*p. 1166*)

50–55. d (*p. 1166*)

50–56. b (*p. 1166*)

50–57. c (*p. 1167*)

50–58. a (*p. 1167*)

CHAPTER 51

51–1. b (*p. 1173*)

51–2. c (*p. 1174*)

51–3. b (*p. 1173*)

51–4. d (*p. 1174*)

51–5. a (*p. 1174*)

51–6. a (*p. 1174*)

51–7. b (*p. 1174*)

51–8. c (*p. 1175*)

51–9. b (*p. 1175*)

51–10. b (*p. 1175*)

51–11. c (*p. 1175*)

51–12. d (*p. 1176*)

51–13. c (*p. 1176*)

51–14. c (*p. 1176*)

51–15. b (*p. 1176*)

51–16. a (*p. 1176*)

51–17. d (*p. 1177*)

51–18. c (*p. 1177*)

51–19. d (*p. 1177*)

51–20. b (*p. 1177*)

51–21. c (*p. 1177*)

51–22. a (*p. 1178*)

51–23. b (*p. 1178*)

51–24. d (*p. 1178*)

51–25. d (*p. 1178*)

51–26. d (*p. 1179*)

51–27. a (*p. 1179*)

51–28. a (*p. 1180*)

51–29. a (*p. 1180*)

51–30. c (*p. 1180*)

51–31. b (*p. 1180*)

51–32. c (*p. 1181*)

51–33. c (*p. 1181*)

51–34. d (*p. 1182*)

51–35. b (*p. 1183*)

51–36. b (*p. 1183*)

51–37. d (*p. 1184*)

51–38. d (*p. 1185*)

51–39. a (*p. 1185*)

51–40. b (*p. 1186*)

51–41. a (*p. 1186*)

51–42. c (*p. 1186*)

51–43. d (*p. 1186*)

51–44. b (*p. 1186*)

51–45. b (*p. 1187*)

51–46. d (*p. 1187*)

51–47. b (*p. 1188*)

51–48. c (*p. 1189*)

51–49. a (*p. 1189*)

51–50. b (*p. 1189*)

51–51. c (*p. 1190*)

51–52. c (*p. 1191*)

51–53. b (*p. 1192*)

51–54. d (*p. 1192*)

51–55. c (*p. 1192*)

51–56. d (*p. 1193*)

51–57. b (*p. 1193*)

51–58. d (*p. 1193*)

51–59. b (*p. 1193*)

51–60. d (*p. 1193*)

51–61. b (*p. 1194*)

51–62. d (*p. 1194*)

51–63. d (*p. 1194*)

51–64. c (*p. 1195*)

51–65. a (*p. 1196*)

51–66. b (*p. 1196*)

51–67. c (*p. 1197*)

51–68. c (*p. 1197*)

CHAPTER 52

52–1. b (*p. 1203*)

52–2. d (*p. 1203*)

52–3. a (*p. 1203*)

52–4. c (*p. 1203*)

52–5. b (*p. 1204*)

52–6. c (*p. 1204*)

52–7. d (*p. 1204*)

52–8. d (*p. 1204*)

52–9. a (*p. 1205*)

52–10. d (*p. 1206*)

52–11. d (*p. 1206*)

52–12. d (*p. 1207*)

52–13. d (*p. 1207*)

52–14. b (*p. 1207*)

52–15. d (*p. 1208*)

52–16. c (*p. 1209*)

52–17. b (*p. 1210*)

52–18. c (*p. 1210*)

52–19. d (*p. 1215*)

52–20. d (*p. 1215*)

52–21. d (*p. 1216*)

52–22. c (*p. 1217*)

52–23. a (*p. 1214*)

52–24. b (*p. 1215*)

52–25. d (*p. 1204*)

52–26. d (*p. 1218*)

52–27. d (*p. 1215*)

52–28. a (*p. 1217*)

52–29. d (*p. 1217*)

CHAPTER 53

53–1. c (*p. 1223*)

53–2. a (*p. 1223*)

53–3. c (*p. 1223*)

53–4. d (*p. 1224*)

53–5. c (*p. 1224*)

53–6. a (*p. 1225*)

53–7. a (*p. 1225*)

53–8. b (*p. 1225*)

53–9. c (*p. 1225*)

53–10. b (*p. 1225*)

53–11. b (*p. 1226*)

53–12. b (*p. 1226*)

53–13. a (*p. 1226*)

53–14. d (*p. 1227*)

53–15. a (*p. 1227*)

53–16. d (*p. 1227*)

53–17. d (*p. 1227*)

53–18. d (*p. 1228*)

53–19. d (*p. 1228*)

53–20. c (*p. 1228*)

53–21. c (*p. 1228*)

53–22. b (*p. 1228*)

53–23. b (*p. 1229*)

53–24. b (*p. 1230*)

53–25. b (*p. 1230*)

53–26. c (*p. 1230*)

53–27. d (*p. 1230*)

53–28. a (*p. 1231*)

53–29. d (*p. 1231*)

53–30. b (*p. 1231*)

53–31. a (*p. 1232*)

53–32. b (*p. 1232*)

53–33. d (*p. 1232*)

53–34. b (*p. 1233*)

53–35. d (*p. 1233*)

53–36. b (*p. 1234*)

53–37. d (*p. 1234*)

53–38. a (*p. 1235*)

53–39. a (*p. 1235*)

53–40. c (*p. 1235*)

CHAPTER 54

54–1. c (*p. 1239*)

54–2. a (*p. 1239*)

54–3. d (*p. 1239*)

54–4. c (*p. 1240*)

54–5. d (*p. 1240*)

54–6. c (*p. 1240*)

54–7. b (*p. 1240*)

54–8. c (*p. 1240*)

54–9. d (*p. 1240*)

54–10. a (*p. 1240*)

54–11. d (*p. 1241*)

54–12. c (*p. 1241*)

54–13. b (*p. 1241*)

54–14. a (*p. 1241*)

54–15. b (*p. 1241*)

54–16. b (*p. 1243*)

54–17. d (*p. 1243*)

54–18. a (*p. 1244*)

54–19. c (*p. 1244*)

54–20. d (*p. 1244*)

54–21. c (*p. 1244*)

54–22. b (*p. 1244*)

54–23. b (*p. 1245*)

54–24. c (*p. 1245*)

54–25. a (*p. 1245*)

54–26. d (*p. 1245*)

54–27. c (*p. 1246*)

54–28. d (*p. 1246*)

54–29. b (*p. 1247*)

54–30. a (*p. 1247*)

54–31. d (*p. 1247*)

54–32. c (*p. 1247*)

54–33. d (*p. 1248*)

54–34. b (*p. 1248*)

54–35. d (*p. 1248*)

54–36. c (*p. 1248*)

54–37. d (*p. 1248*)

54–38. a (*p. 1249*)

54–39. c (*p. 1250*)

54–40. b (*p. 1250*)

54–41. d (*p. 1250*)

54–42. a (*p. 1252*)

CHAPTER 55

55–1. a (*p. 1256*)

55–2. a (*p. 1256*)

55–3. d (*p. 1257*)

55–4. c (*p. 1257*)

55–5. b (*p. 1257*)

55–6. d (*p. 1257*)

55–7. b (*p. 1258*)

55–8. c (*p. 1258*)

55–9. d (*p. 1258*)

55–10. d (*p. 1258*)

55–11. d (*p. 1259*)

55–12. d (*p. 1259*)

55–13. b (*p. 1259*)

55–14. a (*p. 1260*)

55–15. b (*p. 1260*)

55–16. c (*p. 1261*)

55–17. b (*p. 1261*)

55–18. a (*p. 1262*)

55–19. a (*p. 1262*)

55–20. b (*p. 1262*)

55–21. c (*p. 1262*)

55–22. b (*p. 1263*)

55–23. c (*p. 1263*)

55–24. c (*p. 1263*)

55–25. b (*p. 1264*)

55–26. d (*p. 1264*)

55–27. a (*p. 1264*)

55–28. d (*p. 1264*)

55–29. d (*p. 1264*)

55–30. a (*p. 1265*)

55–31. b (*p. 1265*)

55–32. a (*p. 1267*)

55–33. d (*p. 1266*)

55–34. b (*p. 1266*)

55–35. d (*p. 1267*)

55–36. c (*p. 1267*)

55–37. b (*p. 1268*)

55–38. d (*p. 1269*)

CHAPTER 56

56–1. d (*p. 1273*)

56–2. b (*p. 1274*)

56–3. c (*p. 1273*)

56–4. a (*p. 1274*)

56–5. a (*p. 1274*)

56–6. a (*p. 1276*)

56–7. b (*p. 1276*)

56–8. d (*p. 1277*)

56–9. c (*p. 1277*)

56–10. c (*p. 1277*)

56–11. d (*p. 1277*)

56–12. c (*p. 1278*)

CHAPTER 57

57–1. b (*p. 1281*)

57–2. c (*p. 1281*)

57–3. c (*p. 1281*)

57–4. a (*p. 1281*)

57–5. a (*p. 1282*)

57–6. a (*p. 1282*)

57–7. b (*p. 1283*)

57–8. c (*p. 1283*)

57–9. c (*p. 1285*)

57–10. c (*p. 1284*)

57–11. a (*p. 1284*)

57–12. d (*p. 1284*)

57–13. b (*p. 1284*)

57–14. a (*p. 1285*)

57–15. c (*p. 1285*)

57–16. b (*p. 1285*)

57–17. c (*p. 1286*)

57–18. d (*p. 1286*)

57–19. b (*p. 1287*)

57–20. d (*p. 1288*)

57–21. d (*p. 1288*)

57–22. c (*p. 1289*)

57–23. d (*p. 1290*)

57–24. b (*p. 1290*)

57–25. a (*p. 1290*)

57–26. c (*p. 1292*)

CHAPTER 58

58–1. b (*p. 1297*)

58–2. b (*p. 1298*)

58–3. b (*p. 1298*)

58–4. b (*p. 1298*)

58–5. c (*p. 1299*)

58–6. a (*p. 1299*)

58–7. b (*p. 1299*)

58–8. b (*p. 1300*)

58–9. d (*p. 1300*)

58–10. d (*p. 1300*)

58–11. a (*p. 1300*)

58–12. b (*p. 1301*)

58–13. d (*p. 1301*)

58–14. c (*p. 1301*)

58–15. c (*p. 1302*)

58–16. d (*p. 1302*)

58–17. a (*p. 1302*)

58–18. d (*p. 1302*)

58–19. a (*p. 1303*)

58–20. b (*p. 1303*)

58–21. d (*p. 1303*)

58–22. c (*p. 1303*)

58–23. c (*p. 1304*)

58–24. a (*p. 1304*)

58–25. d (*p. 1305*)

58–26. c (*p. 1305*)

58–27. a (*p. 1305*)

58–28. a (*p. 1306*)

58–29. c (*p. 1306*)

58–30. b (*p. 1306*)

58–31. c (*p. 1308*)

58–32. b (*p. 1308*)

58–33. a (*p. 1308*)

58–34. d (*p. 1309*)

58–35. c (*p. 1309*)

58–36. b (*p. 1309*)

58–37. a (*p. 1309*)

58–38. d (*p. 1309*)

58–39. c (*p. 1310*)

58–40. b (*p. 1310*)

58–41. c (*p. 1310*)

58–42. d (*p. 1310*)

58–43. d (*p. 1310*)

58–44. c (*p. 1311*)

CHAPTER 59

59–1. c (*p. 1317*)

59–2. d (*p. 1317*)

59–3. c (*p. 1317*)

59–4. a (*p. 1317*)

59–5. c (*p. 1317*)

59–6. a (*p. 1317*)

59–7. d (*p. 1318*)

59–8. d (*p. 1318*)

59–9. c (*p. 1319*)

59–10. a (*p. 1319*)

59–11. c (*p. 1319*)

59–12. d (*p. 1320*)

59–13. d (*p. 1320*)

59–14. c (*p. 1320*)

59–15. d (*p. 1320*)

59–16. b (*p. 1320*)

59–17. c (*p. 1320*)

59–18. b (*p. 1320*)

59–19. b (*p. 1321*)

59–20. d (*p. 1321*)

59–21. a (*p. 1321*)

59–22. d (*p. 1321*)

59–23. c (*p. 1321*)

59–24. c (*p. 1321*)

59–25. d (*p. 1321*)

59–26. a (*p. 1322*)

59–27. a (*p. 1322*)

59–28. c (*p. 1322*)

59–29. a (*p. 1322*)

59–30. d (*p. 1322*)

59–31. a (*p. 1323*)

59–32. b (*p. 1323*)

59–33. b (*p. 1323*)

59–34. d (*p. 1323*)

59–35. b (*p. 1323*)

59–36. c (*p. 1324*)

59–37. d (*p. 1324*)

59–38. a (*p. 1324*)

59–39. a (*p. 1324*)

59–40. b (*p. 1325*)

59–41. c (*p. 1325*)

59–42. a (*p. 1325*)

59–43. d (*p. 1326*)

59–44. c (*p. 1326*)

59–45. d (*p. 1326*)

59–46. a (*p. 1327*)

59–47. b (*p. 1327*)

59–48. a (*p. 1327*)

59–49. c (*p. 1327*)

59–50. c (*p. 1328*)

59–51. c (*p. 1328*)

59–52. b (*p. 1328*)

59–53. c (*p. 1328*)

59–54. b (*p. 1328*)

59–55. c (*p. 1329*)

59–56. b (*p. 1330*)

59–57. a (*p. 1331*)

59–58. a (*p. 1331*)

59–59. d (*p. 1332*)

59–60. b (*p. 1332*)

59–61. c (*p. 1332*)

59–62. a (*p. 1333*)

59–63. b (*p. 1333*)

59–64. a (*p. 1333*)

CHAPTER 60

60–1. c (*p. 1339*)

60–2. a (*p. 1339*)

60–3. b (*p. 1341*)

60–4. d (*p. 1342*)

60–5. b (*p. 1342*)

60–6. b (*p. 1342*)

60–7. d (*p. 1343*)

60–8. d (*p. 1343*)

60–9. c (*p. 1345*)

60–10. c (*p. 1345*)

60–11. d (*p. 1346*)

60–12. c (*p. 1346*)

60–13. d (*p. 1346*)

60–14. a (*p. 1347*)

60–15. c (*p. 1348*)

60–16. a (*p. 1348*)

60–17. c (*p. 1349*)

60–18. a (*p. 1350*)

60–19. a (*p. 1350*)

60–20. d (*p. 1351*)

60–21. a (*p. 1351*)

60–22. c (*p. 1352*)

60–23. c (*p. 1353*)

60–24. b (*p. 1354*)

60–25. **b** (*p. 1356*)

60–26. **d** (*p. 1356*)

CHAPTER 61

61–1. **c** (*p. 1361*)

61–2. **a** (*p. 1361*)

61–3. **c** (*p. 1361*)

61–4. **c** (*p. 1361*)

61–5. **b** (*p. 1362*)

61–6. **d** (*p. 1363*)

61–7. **d** (*p. 1365*)

61–8. **b** (*p. 1365*)

61–9. **c** (*p. 1364*)

61–10. **d** (*p. 1366*)

61–11. **d** (*p. 1365*)

61–12. **a** (*p. 1369*)

61–13. **a** (*p. 1370*)

61–14. **d** (*p. 1370*)

61–15. **a** (*p. 1371*)

61–16. **b** (*p. 1371*)

61–17. **c** (*p. 1371*)

CHAPTER 62

62–1. **d** (*p. 1375*)

62–2. **b** (*p. 1375*)

62–3. **c** (*p. 1356*)

62–4. **b** (*p. 1376*)

62–5. **d** (*p. 1378*)

62–6. **b** (*p. 1378*)

62–7. **d** (*p. 1378*)

62–8. **b** (*p. 1379*)

62–9. **d** (*p. 1379*)

62–10. **c** (*p. 1379*)

62–11. **a** (*p. 1380*)

62–12. **d** (*p. 1380*)

62–13. **c** (*p. 1380*)

Index

The numbers following each entry indicate chapter and question numbers.

Instructions for Obtaining CME

On the following pages are 100 test questions. Please indicate your answers to these questions on the blue answer grid that appears at the end of the book. ANSWERS MUST BE RECORDED IN PENCIL. Complete the CME evaluation form printed on the reverse side. Enclose the completed answer grid and CME evaluation form in the preaddressed envelope along with a check for $20 payable to The University of Texas Southwestern Medical Center at Dallas.

Statement of Educational Need

This study guide was designed to give the reader an understanding of the management of normal and abnormal pregnancies based on sound obstetrical practice, which is presented in detail in *Williams Obstetrics: 20th Edition*. The purpose of this study guide is to assess comprehension and retention of materials covered in the textbook.

In recent years, new data have added substantially to our knowledge of obstetrics and have changed many management schemes and practice patterns. This updated information needs to be disseminated to physicians in order to help improve recognition and management of common obstetrical problems.

Target Audience and Suggested Use of Materials

The said educational material is comprised of the study guide for the 20th edition of *Williams Obstetrics*. It is suggested that, prior to taking the examination, the participants review the 20th edition of *Williams*, complete the questions contained in the study guide, and finally complete the test evaluation.

Educational Objectives

After reviewing the above materials, individuals will be able to:
1. Determine their fund of knowledge with regard to basic obstetrics.
2. Determine their fund of knowledge with regard to high-risk pregnancies and a variety of medical complications of pregnancy.
3. Be able to assess their knowledge base of common labor problems as well as complications at the time of delivery and postpartum.

Continuing Medical Education Questions

1. Which of the following conditions is more commonly associated with placental abruption?

   a. cocaine
   b. hypertension
   c. preterm prematurely ruptured membranes
   d. cigarette smoking

2. What is the term for the condition where the fetal vessels course through membranes and present at the cervical os?

   a. total placenta previa
   b. marginal placenta previa
   c. partial placenta previa
   d. vasa previa

3. Which of the following represents the threshold for blood volume deficit when compensatory mechanisms become inadequate to maintain cardiac output and blood pressure?

   a. 10%
   b. 15%
   c. 25%
   d. 50%

4. How much will the hematocrit increase after one unit of packed red blood cells (250 mL)?

   a. 1 to 2 vol%
   b. 3 to 4 vol%
   c. 6 to 8 vol%
   d. 10 vol%

5. Which of the following is a potential side effect of the calcium channel blocking agent, nifedipine?

   a. decreased uteroplacental perfusion
   b. hypertension
   c. hypoglycemia
   d. hypocalcemia

6. Antenatal corticosteroid administration given at 24 to 34 weeks will result in a decrease in all but which of the following?

   a. respiratory distress syndrome
   b. periventricular hemorrhage
   c. neonatal death
   d. neonatal infection

7. At what gestational age does perinatal mortality first appreciably increase?

   a. 40.5 weeks
   b. 41 weeks
   c. 42 weeks
   d. 43 weeks

8. Which of the following fetal heart rate patterns is most commonly associated with post-term pregnancies complicated by oligohydramnios?

   a. variable decelerations
   b. late decelerations
   c. early decelerations
   d. tachycardia

9. What percent of fetal growth restriction is secondary to fetal infections?

   a. 10%
   b. 50%
   c. 75%
   d. 90%

10. Which of the following genetic syndromes is generally not associated with fetal growth restriction?

    a. trisomy 13
    b. trisomy 18
    c. trisomy 16
    d. Klinefelter syndrome

11. Which of the following is most likely to be associated with a growth-restricted fetus?

    a. antiphospholipid antibodies
    b. maternal anemia
    c. Turner syndrome
    d. maternal weight of 125 lb

12. Which of the following is not a risk factor for fetal macrosomia?

    a. male fetus
    b. previous infant more than 4000 g
    c. maternal smoking
    d. maternal weight of 300 lb

13. Which of the following is the most important risk factor for macrosomia?

    a. multiparity
    b. prolonged gestation
    c. male fetus
    d. diabetes

14. Approximately what percentage of twins present as cephalic-breech?

    a. 1
    b. 27
    c. 75
    d. 90

15. Which of the following is associated with an increase in monozygotic twins?

    a. race
    b. parity
    c. maternal age
    d. none of the above

16. Which of the following complications are reported to be associated with vascular communications in twin gestations?

    a. microcephaly
    b. porencephaly
    c. cerebral palsy
    d. all of the above

17. Chromosomal anomalies are identified in approximately what percentage of early spontaneous abortions?

    a. 1
    b. 10
    c. 50
    d. 99

18. What percentage of Down syndrome is caused by trisomy 21?

    a. 1
    b. 10
    c. 25
    d. 95

19. Which of the following genetic conditions is related to paternal age?

    a. Down syndrome
    b. Turner syndrome
    c. trisomy 13
    d. achondroplasia

20. High doses of which of the following vitamins should be avoided during pregnancy?

    a. vitamin A
    b. folic acid
    c. vitamin C
    d. vitamin D

21. Approximately what percentage of the caucasian population carries a gene for cystic fibrosis?

    a. <1
    b. 4
    c. 25
    d. 80

22. Which of the following anomalies has been associated with chorionic villus sampling?

    a. cleft lip
    b. limb deficit
    c. cardiac deficit
    d. neural tube defect

23. Which of the following is the most common nongenetic cause of mental retardation?

    a. alcohol
    b. cocaine
    c. amphetamines
    d. heroin

24. Which of the following is not associated with an increase in malformations?

    a. vitamin A excess
    b. isotretinoin
    c. etretinate
    d. beta-carotene

25. Which of the following anticonvulsants is associated with a 1 to 2 percent incidence of neural tube defects?

    a. phenobarbital
    b. carbamazapine
    c. phenytoin
    d. valproic acid

26. What percentage of cerebral palsy cases are associated with mental retardation?

    a. 1
    b. 10
    c. 25
    d. 99

27. What percentage of facial nerve palsies are associated with forceps delivery?

    a. 5
    b. 18
    c. 70
    d. 95

28. What percentage of cases of brachial plexus injury follows uneventful vaginal delivery?

    a. 5
    b. 10
    c. 20
    d. over 50

29. Which of the following best defines a reactive nonstress test (NST)?

    a. 1 acceleration of 15 beats/min in 30 min
    b. 2 or more accelerations of 15 beats/min in 20 min
    c. 4 or more accelerations of 15 beats/min in 30 min
    d. 5 or more accelerations of 15 beats/min in 40 min

30. What is the most likely interpretation of a biophysical profile score of 0 to 2?

    a. almost certain fetal asphyxia
    b. probably fetal asphyxia
    c. possible fetal asphyxia
    d. nonasphyxiated normal infant

31. Which of the following is not a component of a basic ultrasound examination during the first trimester?

    a. gestational sac location
    b. amniotic fluid volume
    c. fetal heart motion
    d. fetal number

32. How early is fetal heart activity generally detected by abdominal ultrasound scanning?

    a. 2 weeks
    b. 4 weeks
    c. 7 weeks
    d. 10 weeks

33. A dangling choroid plexus is suggestive of which of the following?

    a. choroid plexus cyst
    b. anencephaly
    c. encephalocele
    d. hydrocephalus

34. What is the estimated risk of childhood leukemia following exposure to 1 to 2 rads of ionizing radiation?

    a. 1 in 20
    b. 1 in 200
    c. 1 in 2000
    d. 1 in 200,000

35. What is the average fetal exposure from a single plain abdominal film?

    a. 100 mrad
    b. 1 to 2 rads
    c. 5 rads
    d. 7 to 8 rads

36. What is the normal colloid oncotic pressure (COP) at term?

    a. 1 mm Hg
    b. 5 mm Hg
    c. 10 mm Hg
    d. 23 mm Hg

37. Which of the following organisms causes toxic shock syndrome?

    a. Bacteroides species
    b. anaerobic Streptococcus
    c. *Escherichia coli*
    d. *Staphylococcus aureus*

38. What percentage of blunt trauma cases are associated with uterine rupture?

    a. less than 1
    b. 20
    c. 50
    d. 70

39. Which of the following is a symptom of heart disease?

    a. progressive dyspnea
    b. syncope with exertion
    c. chest pain
    d. all of the above

40. What is the New York Heart Association classification for a woman with symptoms of cardiac insufficiency at rest?

    a. I
    b. II
    c. III
    d. IV

41. Which of the following cardiac conditions is associated with a maternal mortality approaching 50%?

    a. atrial septal defect
    b. pulmonary hypertension
    c. ventricular septal defect
    d. patent ductus arteriosus

42. How much is vital capacity increased during pregnancy?

    a. 100 to 200 mL
    b. 400 mL
    c. 1000 mL
    d. no increase

43. What is the mortality in pregnant women treated with anticoagulants for pulmonary embolism?

    a. 3%
    b. 12%
    c. 18%
    d. 23%

44. What percentage of pregnant women with asymptomatic bacteriuria will develop pyelonephritis if not treated?

    a. 1
    b. 5
    c. 25
    d. 50

45. Which of the following is a complication associated with parental nutrition?

    a. pneumothorax
    b. hemothorax
    c. brachial plexus injury
    d. all are complications

46. To which FDA category do the drugs cimetidine and ranitidine belong?

    a. A
    b. B
    c. D
    d. X

47. Which of the following chronic conditions is associated with anemia?

    a. renal disease
    b. inflammatory bowel disease
    c. granulomatous infections
    d. all of the above

48. Which of the following is a side effect of erythropoietin treatment during pregnancy?

    a. hypertension
    b. fever
    c. thrombosis
    d. hemolysis

49. What is the incidence of malformation in offspring of mothers with overt diabetes?

    a. 1%
    b. 5 to 10%
    c. 25%
    d. 38%

50. Which of the following conditions are increased in the neonate of mothers with overt diabetes?

    a. hypoglycemia
    b. hypocalcemia
    c. hyperbilirubinemia
    d. all of the above

51. Methimazole used to treat hyperthyroidism during pregnancy may cause which of the following fetal conditions?

   a. aplasia cutis
   b. hyperthyroidism
   c. agranulocytosis
   d. anemia

52. Preterm labor is more common in which of the following syndromes?

   a. Marfan syndrome
   b. Ehlers–Danlos syndrome
   c. rheumatoid arthritis
   d. none of the above

53. Which of the following conditions has the worst prognosis during pregnancy?

   a. polyarteritis nodosa
   b. Marfan syndrome
   c. rheumatoid arthritis
   d. systemic lupus erythematosus

54. Lithium may cause which of the following?

   a. cleft lip
   b. limb defect
   c. Epstein anomaly
   d. neonatal depression

55. What percentage of pregnant women on anticonvulsant therapy will have a child with a congenital malformation?

   a. 3
   b. 14
   c. 28
   d. 39

56. What is melasma?

   a. areolae pigmentation
   b. linea alba pigmentation
   c. face pigmentation
   d. inner thigh pigmentation

57. What is an epulis of pregnancy?

   a. overgrowth of gum capillaries
   b. a melanocytic nevi
   c. a pyogenic granuloma
   d. granuloma gravidarum

58. To which class of drugs does cyclophosphamide belong?

   a. antimetabolites
   b. antibiotics
   c. alkylating agents
   d. folic acid antagonists

59. Approximately how many American women will eventually be afflicted with breast carcinoma?

   a. 1 in 2
   b. 1 in 10
   c. 1 in 100
   d. 1 in 1000

60. What percentage of pregnant women are immune to varicella?

   a. 5 to 10
   b. 25 to 50
   c. 70
   d. 90

61. Which of the following viral infections is associated with a characteristic "slapped cheek" appearance?

   a. rubella
   b. parvovirus
   c. rubeola
   d. influenza

62. Which of the following organisms may cause a "toxic shock-like" syndrome?

   a. group A streptococcus
   b. group B streptococcus
   c. enterococcus
   d. listeria

63. What is the treatment for trichomonas infections in the third trimester of pregnancy?

   a. miconazole
   b. metronidazole
   c. clotrimazole
   d. gantrisin

64. What percentage of women will conceive if no contraception is used for one year?

   a. 10
   b. 25
   c. 50
   d. 90

65. Which of the following is the bioactive estrogen in oral contraceptives?

   a. ethinyl estradiol
   b. mestranol
   c. estriol
   d. estradiol-17β

66. Which of the following intrauterine devices (IUD) is no longer available?

   a. Progestasert
   b. Dalkon shield
   c. levonorgestrel
   d. Copper T 380A

67. What is the average menstrual blood loss with the Progestasert IUD?

   a. 5 mL
   b. 25 mL
   c. 150 mL
   d. 350 mL

68. What tubal sterilization procedure involves crushing a knuckle of tube and ligation with a nonabsorbable suture without resection?

   a. Pomeroy
   b. Parkland
   c. Madlener
   d. Irving

69. What percentage of pregnancies after electrocoagulation are ectopic?

   a. 1
   b. 10
   c. 50
   d. 100

70. Which of the following would be classified as an indirect maternal death?

   a. postpartum hemorrhage
   b. sepsis
   c. mitral stenosis
   d. automobile accident

71. Human chorionic gonadotropin (hCG) is produced exclusively by which of the following tissues?

   a. cytotrophoblast
   b. syncytiotrophoblast
   c. amnion
   d. decidua

72. Which of the following pelvic measurements cannot be measured directly but is computed?

   a. true conjugate
   b. obstetrical conjugate
   c. posterior sagittal diameter of outlet
   d. transverse diameter of the outlet

73. What day of the menstrual cycle would you expect to see the FSH surge?

   a. 5
   b. 10
   c. 14
   d. 18

74. What embryonic layer becomes the avascular fetal membrane?

   a. chorion laeve
   b. decidual membranalis
   c. decidual basalis
   d. decidua parietalis

75. How do you classify human pregnancy?

   a. hypoprogesteronemic
   b. hypergonadotropic
   c. hypoestrogenic
   d. hyperestrogenic

76. Which of the following fetal immunoglobulins is produced in response to infection?

   a. IgA
   b. IgG
   c. IgE
   d. IgM

77. At what stage of gestation does arterial blood pressure reach its nadir?

   a. 10 weeks
   b. 20 weeks
   c. 40 weeks
   d. immediately postpartum

78. What one factor has done more to save mothers' lives than any other factor?

   a. prenatal care
   b. β-mimetics
   c. fetal monitoring
   d. cesarean section

79. Which of the following is not a predisposing factor for a transverse lie?

a. multiparity
b. placenta previa
c. oligohydramnios
d. uterine anomalies

80. What enzyme is responsible for phosphorylation of myosin?

a. tubulinase
b. contractionase
c. myosin light chain kinase
d. cAMP-dependent protein kinase

81. What is the presentation if Leopold maneuvers reveal (1) breech in fundus, (2) resistant plane to mother's left flank, (3) head movable, and (4) cephalic prominence on the maternal right?

a. ROT
b. LOT
c. ROA
d. LOA

82. What is the ritgen maneuver?

a. complete breech extraction
b. flexion of maternal legs to abdomen
c. forceful turning of anterior shoulder laterally
d. forward pressure on the fetal chin through the perineum

83. Which of the following is NOT a criterion possibly linking intrapartum events to birth asphyxia and cerebral palsy?

a. umbilical artery pH <7.0
b. Apgar score 3 at 10 min
c. sepsis
d. seizures in the neonate

84. What is the most common side effect from intraepidural opiates?

a. pruritis
b. urinary retention
c. nausea and vomiting
d. headaches

85. An increase in pCO_2 of 20 will lower the umbilical artery pH by what degree?

a. 0.04 units
b. 0.08 units
c. 0.16 units
d. 0.32 units

86. What is the definition of dystocia?

a. precipitous labor
b. normal labor in breech
c. labor in a woman with prior cesarean section
d. abnormal progress in labor

87. Which of the following would decrease the likelihood of successful external cephalic version?

a. amniotic fluid index of 10 cm
b. maternal weight of 240 lb
c. posterior placenta location
d. breech at $+1$ station

88. What is the increased incidence of cord prolapse in a woman with a contracted pelvis?

a. no increase
b. 1 to 2 times
c. 4 to 6 times
d. 8 to 10 times

89. Which forceps has a sliding lock?

a. Barton
b. Kielland
c. Tucker–McLane
d. Simpsons

90. Which of the following is significantly different when frank breech vaginal deliveries are compared to those delivered by cesarean section?

a. Apgar scores
b. hospital stay
c. cord blood gas analysis
d. no differences

91. Which of the following are associated with increasing the cesarean section rate during the past two decades?

a. electronic fetal monitoring
b. breech presentation
c. malpractice litigation
d. all of the above

92. By conventional definition, the puerperium is from birth until what week postpartum?

    a. 2 weeks
    b. 4 weeks
    c. 6 weeks
    d. 12 weeks

93. What is the treatment of choice for necrotizing fasciitis?

    a. antibiotics
    b. surgical debridement
    c. antibiotics and surgical debridement
    d. antibiotics, surgical debridement, and heparin

94. Which of these pregnancy complications does not increase significantly with advanced maternal age?

    a. previa/abruption
    b. diabetes
    c. hypertension
    d. low birthweight

95. What is the most common cause of first trimester abortions?

    a. infection
    b. chromosomal abnormalities
    c. antiphospholipid antibody syndrome
    d. chronic maternal disease

96. What is the leading cause of maternal mortality during the first trimester?

    a. ectopic pregnancy
    b. septic abortion
    c. embolism
    d. anesthesia complications

97. Which of the following female genital mutilation procedures consists of removal of the clitoris, labia minora, and at least two thirds of the labia majora?

    a. circumcision
    b. sunna
    c. excision
    d. infibulation

98. At what week of pregnancy does acute hydramnios tend to develop?

    a. 16 to 20 weeks
    b. 24 to 28 weeks
    c. 32 to 34 weeks
    d. >36 weeks

99. What is the most common physical finding in women with molar pregnancy?

    a. tachycardia
    b. ovarian masses
    c. size greater than dates
    d. hypertension

100. Which of the following is NOT associated with HELLP syndrome?

    a. hemolysis
    b. abnormal liver functions
    c. hemoconcentration
    d. low platelets